Essays on
Nursing Leadership

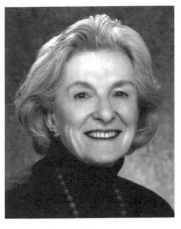

Claire M. Fagin, PhD, RN, FAAN, is a consultant to foundations, developing national programs, and educational institutions. Dr. Fagin's career has blended an interest in consumer health issues with professional health and nursing isssues. She is known for her efforts with consumers and health professionals to create a new paradigm for access and quality. She served as dean of the School of Nursing at the University of Pennsylvania from January 1977 to January 1992, and as the Interim President of the University from July 1, 1993 to June 30, 1994. Dr. Fagin was the first woman to serve as Chief Executive Officer of the University and the first woman to serve a term as Interim President of any Ivy League University. Presently she is Director of the John A. Hartford Foundation program "Building Academic Geriatric Nursing Capacity."

Dr. Fagin has served on three corporate boards (Provident Mutual, and Salomon, Inc. and is currently on Radian Guarantee, Inc.), and has been in elected and appointed positions with many professional organizations. Currently she is a member of the Board of the Van Ameringen Foundation, the Visiting Nurse Service of New York, the New York Academy of Medicine, and is a member or Fellow of the Institute of Medicine, National Academy of Sciences; the American Academy of Nursing; the Expert Panel on Nursing of the World Health Organization; and the American Academy of Arts and Sciences.

Dr. Fagin has received ten honorary doctoral degrees and numerous alumni, civic, and professional awards. In recognition of her contribution to nursing education and leadership and her influence on health care policy, Dr. Fagin received the Honorary Recognition Award of the American Nurses Association, the most prestigious honor awarded in the nursing profession. Among her other awards are the first Distinguished Scholar Award given by the American Nurses Foundation, and the Hildegard E. Peplau Award (for her work in psychiatric nursing), from the American Nurses Association. In Fall 1998 Dr. Fagin was made a "Living Legend" by the American Academy of Nursing and received the President's Medal from New York University.

Essays on
Nursing Leadership

Claire M. Fagin, PhD, RN, FAAN

Springer Publishing Company

Copyright © 2000 by Springer Publishing Company, Inc.

Springer Publishing Company, Inc.
536 Broadway
New York, NY 10012-3955

Acquisitions Editor: Ruth Chasek
Production Editor: Helen Song
Cover design by Susan Hauley

00 01 02 03 04 / 5 4 3 2 1

Library of Congress Cataloging-in-Publication Data

Fagin, Claire M.
    Essays on nursing leadership / Claire Fagin.
        p. ; cm.
    Includes bibliographical references and index.
    ISBN 0-8261-1357-5 (hardcover)
    1. Nursing services—Administration.   2. Leadership.   I. Title.
    [DNLM: 1. Fagin, Claire M. 2. Nursing—Essays. 3. Education,
Nursing—Essays.   4. Leadership—Essays. WY 16 F155e 2000]
    RT89 .F34 2000
    362.1'73'068—dc21   00-030055
                                                                             CIP

For Sam,

my even keel

Contents

Contributors

Leah F. Binder, MGA, MA
Executive Director
Health Community Coaliton
Farmington, Maine

Donna Diers, RN, MSN, FAAN
Annie W. Goodrich Professor of Nursing
Yale University
New Haven, Connecticut

Suzanne Gordon
Journalist
Author of *Life Support: Three Nurses on the Front Lines*

Joan E. Lynaugh, PhD, FAAN
Emeritus Professor and Term Chair
History of Nursing and Health Care
School of Nursing
University of Pennylvania

Foreword

Nursing is, at its core, a practice discipline. While nurses have forged successful careers in many and varied roles in health care, their legitimacy and versatility derives, in large part, from nursing's clinical care base. Indeed, nurses as a group enjoy a level of social prestige not accorded to other occupations with comparable average educational attainment, because of their commitment, paraphrasing Virginia Henderson's definition of nursing, to do for patients what they would do for themselves if they were able.

Paradoxically, the very attributes that have gained nurses prestige and societal respect have perceived derogatory connotations and implications. Nurses' status derives in large part from their association with a type of work that many in society shy away from.

In addition to the special status nurses derive from the "laying on of hands," the profession also derives enhanced social prestige from its close partnership with physicians in the provision of science-based medical treatments. But, nurses have long chaffed under the subordination to physicians that characterizes relations between the two professions. Herein lies what Eliot Friedson (1970, p. 66) describes as nursing's curious dilemma:

> "To escape subordination to medical authority, [nursing] must find some area of work over which it can claim and maintain a monopoly, but it must do so in a setting in which the central task is healing and controlled by medicine."

In the following book, Claire Fagin writes about some of nursing's missteps as the profession sought to resolve this "curious" dilemma. The most serious of these missteps were academic nursing's retreat from its clinical care base and its isolation from physicians. The goal of moving nursing education from the apprentice system of hospital-sponsored nursing schools that trained most nurses through 1970 to mainstream institutions of higher education was a good one. Nursing did pay a price, however, for the "withdrawal" of much of its leadership into academia. Among Claire Fagin's many contributions to contemporary nursing, none is more important than her leadership in the reunification of nursing education and practice, and improved nurse/physician collaboration.

Many of the essays in this book provide the rationale for the reunification of nursing education and practice, and discuss general and specific strategies for achieving it. The integration of practice with education and research is key to advancing the state of nursing science and improving the effectiveness of nursing practice. As we enter the 21st century, it is increasingly clear that one of the greatest challenges to university nursing schools will be to bring the status and authority of academic nursing leadership to bear on influencing the practice setting for nurses as the health care system undergoes fundamental change.

Linda H. Aiken, PhD, FAAN, FRCN
Philadelphia, Pennsylvania

REFERENCES

Fox, R. C., Aiken, L. H., & Messikomer, C. M. (1990). The culture of caring: AIDS and the nursing profession. *The Milbank Quarterly, 68,* 226–256.

Friedson, E. (1970). *Professional dominances: The social structure of medical care.* Chicago: Aldine Publishing Company.

Henderson, V. (1966). *The nature of nursing: A definition and its implications for practice, research, and education.* New York: Macmillan Co.

Hughes, E. C. (1958). *Twenty thousand nurses tell their story.* Philadelphia: J. B. Lippincott.

Scott, R. A., Aiken, L. H., Mechanic, D., & Moravscik, J. (1995). Organizational aspects of caring. *Milbank Quarterly, 73,* 77–95.

Foreword

Perhaps no leader has been a more astute and passionate voice for the nursing profession in national health policy discussions than Claire M. Fagin. This rich selection of her works reflects the progression of her thoughts about health policy and nursing's proper place in it over the past two decades. For better or worse, the themes and topics of these papers are still extremely timely today.

Probably more than any other profession, nursing is suited to provide the transformational leaders that will bring us successfully to health care for the next millennium. Additionally, nursing's health and wellness paradigm is "in style," because for the first time ever the economic incentives in health care encourage and reward providers to prevent illness, and keep people out of expensive in-patient settings. The problem is that the businessmen and physicians currently leading the managed care parade are guiding the change according to the same old medical model of disease and treatment, where the entirety of our focus is on people only after they are already sick. As Abraham Maslow put it, "when you're a carpenter, the only tools you know how to use are a hammer and a nail." Yet, in the new world of managed care a hammer and a nail are not going to work any longer.

During the span of time in which these papers were produced, health care has taken a sharp turn in a very different direction. Health care as most of us have known it for years is gone forever. Currently, in "a very distinctively American fashion" (as the PEW Health Professions Report put it), we are seeing raging market-driven reform. Indeed, there is a very unapologetic emphasis on margins of profit, competition, and consolidation to achieve strength in the marketplace.

As Uwe Rinehardt said at a recent New York Academy of Medicine meeting, we are a "bunch of hard asses" as a nation. We had the opportunity to enact reforms that would provide care to all Americans and we rejected it in favor of market-driven reforms that continue to leave millions of Americans without care.

True, the jury is still out on the new world of managed care; its long term assets and liabilities remain to be seen, but one thing is certain: Quality issues loom more heavily on the minds of consumers and policy makers every day. Many observers believe that quality of care will be the most crucial issue for us in the future.

Dr. Fagin was notably the first practitioner in the nation to convene health care professionals to address the quality issue—in a symposium entitled *The Abandonment of the Patient*. Testimonials were offered by patients who had recently had atrocious experiences, providers talked of downsizing and severe nursing cutbacks. One nursing administrator spoke candidly about the dangerous nurse to patient ratios in her institution, in the range of 3–4 nurses for 25–26 very sick patients. Many pointed out the obvious link between deteriorating quality of care and the wholesale cutbacks in the nursing staff. It was also pointed out that for fear of loss of jobs, nurses often refrain from speaking up about poor quality practices that put patients' well-being in jeopardy.

And yet, if nurses don't speak out about poor quality issues, who will? Reports about egregious practices on the part of Managed Care Organizations are rampant. News stories on the refusal to treat critically ill newborns, casualties due to outmoded dialysis equipment, lack of timely claims payment, and lack of continuity of care appear daily in the headlines.

Quality concerns should not cause us, however, to lose sight of the extraordinary opportunity in the new managed care environment for nursing. Nursing's vision of a comprehensive approach to care is the most appropriate approach to delivering care and now the most economically rewarding. Physicians and managed care executives are well aware of what's needed—but they don't know how to do it. I chuckle when I hear physician friends talk about the need for a "biopsychosocial" model of care. That's what they called my under-graduate curriculum 25 years ago!

Nursing alone has the biological, the psychosocial, and the popula-tion perspectives to provide the leadership that is needed to manage the care of populations; to keep them well and prevent illness in addition to managing chronic illness. The nursing profession can fix what ails the managed care system—because what ails it is this: we have a huge biomedical enterprise that has been challenged to shift its focus from curing the disease to preventing it in the first place. And the chief architects of the system have no idea how to go about it. But nurses do. At long last it seems the health care delivery system is ready to reward the approaches to patient care nursing has always advocated.

But unless the nursing profession is psychologically prepared to play a leadership role and unless nursing education can prepare nurses for leadership roles in the future managed care environment, this golden opportunity will be lost. Graduates of our programs enter a world dominated and fueled by Wall Street and Washington and they know little or nothing about it. Yet nurses are, in terms of their knowledge, skills and competencies, extremely well suited to be the primary care providers, the case managers, and the educators in the new managed care system. It's time for the nursing profession to take a hard look at itself and reinvent itself for the future, just as medicine and the others are being forced to do under managed care. None of us will be spared by the white water changes ahead.

This collection of works will lend valuable insights into these current challenges—insights from one of the masters. These works from Claire Fagin's brilliant career and the wisdom of those experi-ences will perhaps assist nursing at this time, to rise to its true place at the helm of health care, so that people's well-being, not just profit margins, will determine the future. I personally want to thank Claire for making this collection available so that many more will be inspired by her, as I, and many others have been.

Pamela J. Maraldo, PhD, RN, FAAN
New York, New York

Preface

This book represents a small selection of my writings over a period of 30+ years. Included are previously published pieces as well as some essays and articles, which are published here for the first time. I have tried to select those papers among my writings that demonstrate the wonderful diversity possible in a nursing career and that speak to contemporary issues and problems. Some of the previously published works have been edited so that data is as current as possible without altering the integrity of the original article.

My editor, Ruth Chasek, Ursula Springer, and I used two criteria for selection of the contents. One was to choose those writings that had the most to say to today's nurses. The other was to nurture the enormous potential for leadership in nursing, both within the profession and in the health care arena. I hope that some of what I have learned in my career can be passed down to a new generation of nurses.

An overarching characteristic of my work has been communication about nursing in order to influence policy within the profession and politically. Communication of issues from the standpoint of where we have been, where we are, and where we need to be and how to get there, seems to be a central theme of my writings for a nursing audience. Communication about nursing—its problems and potential—and positioning it in the health field for professionals in other disciplines, and for consumers, is another theme of this overarching characteristic.

Nursing, as my friend and colleague Gretta Styles has said, is what nurses do. Professional nursing, as Martha Rogers said, is what nurses know. Putting what you know into what you do allows nurses to develop the most flexible career patterns of any group I have observed. The flexibility is provided by the extent to which the informed behavior can influence our interactions with the individual patient, groups of patients and families, communities, and policy making groups. My experiences are only one example of the myriad opportunities nurses can have or create for themselves.

One aspect of a nursing career that may not be expressed sufficiently in this book is the extraordinary colleagueship that many of us have experienced. Although many of the articles appearing in the book could have been received with anger and hostility because they challenged the status quo, the reception was quite different. Surely there were many people who did not care much for my solutions, particularly to educational entry issues. Nonetheless, I have received love and affirmation from my colleagues, more often than not.

I hope that this book will help others, both nurses and non-nurses, understand the nature of nursing and a nursing career.

Claire M. Fagin
New York, New York
2000

CHAPTER ONE

Author Profile: About Claire Fagin

Until I was in high school, my stated ambition was to be a physician—to follow in the footsteps of an extremely successful aunt. I had some inkling by that time that I did not want to be a physician but had not gotten around to breaking the news to my family, whose goals for me had been clear from early childhood. By the end of high school I had become convinced that medicine was not of interest to me, but I had no idea what I would find interesting. I graduated from high school at 16 and enrolled at Hunter College in New York City (still quiet about my rebellion from the family's professional dreams for me) in a rigorous program that would keep my options open. That first semester was wonderful, and my enjoyment of math and languages led me to consider adopting one or the other as a possible major. By the summer of my freshman year, the battlefront news of World War II had become an extremely important part of life, and thoughts of how to serve our country were shared by young men and women. The boys would either enlist or be drafted, while most girls would sit at home and write letters. My need to participate in some way was met in part by active political participation, but that wasn't enough for me. I was not quite 17, and there were not many direct-action opportunities at that age.

Note: Portions of this chapter were published in Schorr, T., and Zimmerman, A., (Eds.), 1988. *Making choices, taking chances: Nurse leaders tell their stories.* St. Louis, MO: C.V. Mosby, 94–104.

I started noticing billboard pictures of gorgeous women in the uniform of the U.S. Cadet Nurse Corps. I thought, "Why not?" This would meet my need to serve, and it might even interest me. I had by then had some contact with nurses in public health, since my next door neighbor was a public health nurse, and my father had been visited by a public health nurse after suffering a myocardial infarction. While not inspiring me in any overt way, they certainly provided a positive image, and I was able to recall that image when I started to consider nursing as a career. A friend and I began to investigate local hospital schools, but before we did anything serious, we happened on the office of the New York City Nursing Council for War Service. The name alone grabbed us, and we went in to see what it was all about. This was my first important career-shaping event, and I will always be grateful to the woman we met that day. Her name was Dorothy Wheeler. (She later became the director of nursing for the Veterans Administration system and was written up in the *New York Times* as the highest paid nurse in the country.)

Miss Wheeler was an inspiration to me and influenced substantially the subsequent course of my career. She was a petite, attractive woman who was extremely alert, perceptive, and vivacious. Her interview with us was sharp and revealing, and her advice was convincing. She told us that under no circumstances should we consider a hospital school of nursing. "The wave of the future is baccalaureate education," she said, adding that no person already in college should dream of going to a hospital school. She sat with us and wrote down three schools she thought we should look into based on the information she had gleaned from the interview. They were Adelphi University, Skidmore College, and Wagner College. We followed Miss Wheeler's advice and interviewed at these schools. For a variety of reasons, we both chose Wagner College. Not the least of those reasons was the fact that Mary Burr, the dean at that time, was a warm, motherly, accepting person who did not question our leaving college at the end of our freshman year.

My experience with Miss Wheeler was the first of many such experiences that I have had in nursing that have directly influenced my future. This type of experience has led me to believe we place too much emphasis on mentoring, that is, the long-term continuing relationship with an influential, and too little on the ad hoc brief counseling experience that many of us have been lucky enough to have. As I look from the present back to that fortunate walk on Lexington Avenue in New York, where I met Miss Wheeler, I can identify many other colleagues, teachers, friends, and family members who have contributed in various ways to my development.

Before I expound on the many experiences I have had in this wonderful profession, here are several constants that have influenced all my work at different levels of leadership:

1. I believe in democratic participation and am most comfortable when there is shared decision making. This belief was fostered by my family. It was reinforced during my time at Wagner College and came into full bloom in my experience and graduate work in psychiatric nursing.

2. The quality of empathy was developed in me by very early experiences in my home, and then later was honed to a great extent by my personal and professional experience with and in psychiatry. My mother's enormous asset (and weakness) was her ability to see the other person's view no matter what her child said. If she couldn't see it immediately, she would ask probing questions that forced me to recognize that I might have had a part in a given situation, whether I was bloodied or not. I hated it, but I know that this interaction taught me empathy. Through this kind of learning, one can build one's interpersonal competence at many points in life. I have built on this personally and have used my mother's technique, with intellectual addendums, in both teaching and administration.

3. The relationships I enjoy most are peer relationships. If people are smarter than I or better at something than I am, I don't feel competitive with them. Rather, I feel inspired to try to learn more, or to copy, or to follow. I have no problem sitting at the feet of experts, if they are truly expert. When people are in the learning stages of life, it is my pleasure to help them realize themselves and their potential. I have no need for nor do I take much pleasure in a superordinate role. As an administrator, this plays out in the standard I use to measure myself: The extent to which I have built leaders around me dictates my success.

4. I am an activist. I have never been able to sit back when faced with real or perceived unfairness. I fight in skirmishes, battles, and wars. Little did I know when I chose this provocative profession that this characteristic would be exercised so often.

Does it seem strange that these four constants have played a major part at every crossroad in my work life? Perhaps it explains to some extent why the nursing profession, which was such an accidental career choice for me, has met my personal and professional needs and goals better than any other profession I can imagine. In a career that now spans 50 years, there has been plenty of time for such reflection. It has been said that many nurses do not have a dream of how their careers will unfold. That certainly is true for me, yet the progression of my career has logical steps in it and more similarity than difference.

FIRST STEPS

I was in the second class of nursing students at Wagner College. The college was welcoming to us, and the student group was diverse and not much different from any other college group. The program was interesting in its plan. The first year was spent on the Wagner campus in Staten Island, New York. During that year we took the requisite sciences, liberal arts, and some nursing courses. The following two years we affiliated in various hospitals, living in nurses' residences and returning to campus one day each week. At the end of the three-year program, we received a diploma in nursing and were eligible to take the state board examinations. A fourth year to complete the liberal arts and science requirements for the BS degree was optional. Because of the war and the number of young men being drafted, Wagner had an innovative program of study with courses offered in one-month blocks. This meant that if a male student was drafted, he would be able to complete the courses in which he had enrolled.

I had no idea how I would fare in the science component of the program, nor did I have the vaguest idea of whether or not I would succeed in or enjoy the nursing courses. As it turned out, I disliked but excelled in the sciences, and I did well in and loved every nursing course. At the end of each specialty component—surgical nursing, medical nursing, pediatric nursing, and operating room nursing—I felt I might choose that particular concentration for my future work role. After a few of these experiences, my confusion was rampant, since it was obvious that I couldn't prefer everything. However, my learning experiences at Creedmoor State Hospital soon solved the dilemma. It became clear very rapidly that I would choose psychiatric nursing for my option during my senior cadet experience and that I would seek a position in that field upon graduation.

Pursuing psychiatric nursing did not turn out to be so easy, since I had to complete my last year at Wagner and since there was no psychiatric hospital nearby. Instead, I worked at Seaview, a long-term tuberculosis hospital, in pediatrics as a staff nurse and later as a clinical instructor. The psychological needs of these children were staggering, given the severity of their illnesses and the long-term separation from their families. Certainly, this experience helped to further my interests in psychiatric nursing (particularly in child psychiatric nursing) and led me to a glimmer of interest in the subject of separation. Some of the colleagues I had at Seaview were friends I had made at Wagner, and others I had met during my affiliation there earlier. So, additional building blocks began to set a foundation for my future. Because this was an understaffed public hospital in a rather remote location (at that time), there was a lot of opportunity for innovation and experimentation in testing the system, in doing as much with patients as we were capable of, and in leadership. I received my BSN in May 1948. By the time I left Seaview in October 1948 (for a system transfer to Bellevue Hospital and adolescent psychiatry), I had tested all of these parameters and felt quite confident in my nursing skills and in my ability to do for patients what was "right" without worrying about bureaucratic restraints. Another turning point was negotiated as I entered a new and, as it turned out, critical, formative experience.

Bellevue was different from Seaview in every way, shape, and form. While also a city hospital, it was reasonably well staffed with nurses, was extremely well staffed with physicians, residents, and interns from prestigious medical schools, and was dominated by the Bellevue mystique. The Bellevue cap was powerful, and at times I thought I would do almost anything to have one. However, I learned again that an eye on the patient and on his needs helps you accomplish your major goals, providing you can tell people what you want and the reason why—even without the Bellevue cap or the MD degree. Leadership can't help but thrive after you have had enough success-ful experiences of that type and have learned what does and does not work.

On my first morning at Bellevue, I met my future supervisor, Mildred Gottdank, the director of education. She was a tiny person with piercing eyes, and she was very verbal, intimidating, tough, challenging, and smart. It was obvious that she knew more about psychiatry than I knew existed, and she had a master's degree. A friend and I had left Seaview together, and we were fortunately together for this first interview with the indomitable Miss Gottdank. We could see at a glance that as she took her long look at us she was thinking, "What on earth do I need you two for?" She said, "Miss Mintzer, you are going to PQ 5. That's our adolescent unit, and you have all this pediatric experience." My friend was assigned to O 7, the unit for disturbed women. Miss Gottdank then walked out of her office with us to deliver us to our assignments. PQ 5 came first. She walked to the door, rang the bell, and opened the door with her key. I walked in, and as she closed the door, I could hear the key turning in the lock. There I stood, terror-struck, surrounded by a mob of adolescent boys who were staring me up and down.

This unit's population was boys between 12 and 16 years old, most of whom had come in from the courts with records ranging from truancy to murder. They were tough in appearance, and many were also tough in behavior. I stood transfixed at the locked door. That was the first test of whether or not I would make it there. Initially, the boys tried to provoke me by flirting and pulling my hair, and they watched to see how I would handle the leaders. It was all hazy to me, but I stood my ground, got through the first day, and went on to what proved to be one of the most satisfying and influential experiences of my life. I worked at Bellevue for two years, loved every minute of it, and could not wait to get out of bed in the morning to rush there. I visited patients and families with other colleagues in my off time and made more lasting relationships than I can recount in this short sketch.

I loved working with adolescents and was always good with them. I worked with a team of psychiatrists, residents, teachers, and psychologists, which taught me what successful colleagueship and interdependence were all about and filled me with a sense of my own worth and the worth of psychiatric nursing. Three of us—one psychiatrist, one vocational psychologist, and I—worked particularly well together. We followed youngsters from the ward to their homes on our own time and worked with their families in prototypic ways that were extremely rewarding to us and very helpful to them. I worked with students from a number of schools, and while the course content was far from sophisticated, I was learning all the time and was a good instructor (according to later reports).

I had some difficulties there with nurses and residents who were more tradition and position bound than quality oriented, but whenever called to explain my behavior to Miss Gottdank, I managed to explain the theory behind my intervention, and she was satisfied and went to bat for me. When the residents complained, it was to the chief psychiatrist, Dr. Paul Zimmering. He was equally supportive of my work and made sure his support of me and of psychiatric nursing was extremely visible at group meetings when new residents were present. So, with all of these good things happening (at $2,400 a year), why did I leave Bellevue?

In May 1949 one of my close nursing colleagues decided to get a master's degree, and she left for Smith College School of Social Work. That gave me some pause to think, since I was education oriented and it was obvious that I could use more grounding in theory to explain what I was doing and what I believed. I talked a great deal in the intuitive mode rather than in the intellectual mode, and that bothered me. Miss Gottdank could interview a patient for 5 minutes and get more information than I could in 45 minutes. That bothered me, too.

In July a new ward instructor joined our group. She had just completed a master's degree at Teachers College and had been in the first class in psychiatric nursing directed by Hildegard Peplau (not yet known by a wide nursing public). This nurse, Gertrude Stokes, was different. When she spoke at our meetings, her comments were more theoretical and intellectual than mine. Naturally, given what I have said earlier, I admired this and wanted to be like her. Until then, I had thought that I was a really terrific speaker. I decided that if I was to stay in this field, I needed to be able to talk the way she and Miss Gottdank did. So, I applied to Teachers College and was awarded a National Institute of Mental Health (NIMH) fellowship to study full-time for my master's degree with Hildegard Peplau. I took a leave of absence from Bellevue, fully expecting to return. This was another major turning point in my life and certainly a building block in my career.

GRADUATE EDUCATION, NEW JOBS, MARRIAGE

Times were really different then for graduate study in nursing. The student body was extremely diverse with a range in age from me at 23 to men and women in their middle to late forties. The courses during that year were superb, and, again, the opportunities for making lasting friendships and colleagueships abounded. In addition to the special experience of learning from Hilda, we met Esther Garrison during that year. Esther was the chief nurse in the training branch at NIMH and was responsible for the development of support for nursing within NIMH. She had a unique way of spotting and encouraging talent and did so with many people, including Hilda Peplau and Gwen Tudor Will, a classmate in my program and already a nursing leader.

Lest anyone get the impression that I was a bold and assertive person at that time, let me dispel that notion. I was rather shy, and asserting myself did not come easily. However, I was a doer and a fighter, so I managed to speak up for issues I believed in, and since I never suffered as much from doing that as from not doing it, eventually I built enough confidence to have such behaviors become part of my persona.

Hilda Peplau and many of my classmates were very affirming and supportive. There was a sense among all of us that we were future leaders, and everything necessary to make this happen was available to us. Some were already in leadership positions, and others were about to be placed in established roles. It was a heady atmosphere, indeed. In addition to Hilda, I had several memorable professors at Teachers College, including Goodwin Watson, Lyman Bryson, Emma Spaney, and others.

When I visited Bellevue to plan for my return, I was told that I would now be a supervisor, since I was overprepared for my previous position. I was crushed because a supervisor at that time was a very traditional role, was unconnected with patient care, and was characterized by the figure of a crisply uniformed nurse going from floor to floor with a clipboard. There was no way that I was going to be a supervisor at Bellevue. And so, another turning point was forced on me. Hilda had developed an outline for a study of the functions and qualifications of psychiatric nurses for the National League for Nursing (which was then the National League of Nursing Education).

She decided that I should be the director of that study and convinced the executive director of the League to interview me. This was an interesting experience. I had been told that the job paid $6,000 per year. During the interview, the executive director asked me how old I was. I told her that I was 24, and she said the job would pay $4,200 per year. When I said I had been told the salary was $6,000, she said that was true, but that I was too young for that salary. I carried on for a good bit about the unfairness of this arrangement, and she said that in six months, if I proved myself, she would give me a raise, which she did—but not up to $6,000. I lost a physician boyfriend over that, since he was clearly after my money.

I assumed the title of psychiatric nurse consultant and directed a study that was to be the first of my publications. I never could have completed it without Hilda and a few other colleagues. I was not a researcher, nor was I a writer. It took many near misses before that document was completed. The term "consultant" was something of a misnomer, and as I traveled all over the United States to gather data for the study, it really got in my way. All the people I interviewed were older and more experienced than I was, and their greetings were often colored by their preconceptions about this young New Yorker with a high falutin' title. It took me a while to get through that, and in some cases I didn't. In a few cities there were nurse educators serving on the planning committee for the study who were extremely warm and welcoming. One of these women was Tirzah Morgan, then at the University of Washington. She was an "original" who was wonderful to me during my League year, and she became a good friend in later years.

One month after I had accepted the job with the League, I met Sam Fagin, an electrical engineer working in the Washington area. We married in February 1952, midway through my contract year. We bought a house in suburban Maryland, and I commuted on weekends. Sam was more than accepting about my work. He understood perfectly that I could not leave the position before it was finished, and we managed quite well during the commuting period. I was already known to a minor extent as Claire Mintzer, but I wanted very much to assume his name as my own feminist statement. All of my married nursing and nonnursing professional acquaintances of the previous era had used their maiden names (including my aunt and all her friends), and I felt I was making a new statement as a married professional woman. So it goes.

During the first months of my new position and before my marriage, Gwen Tudor came to see me in New York. She was preparing for a major new position as chief nurse at the Clinical Center, National Institutes of Health, which was still under construction. She asked me to consider becoming her assistant. She wanted me to develop the psychiatric children's unit and be responsible for in-service education. I hesitated, but it became obvious that this was a fabulous opportunity, and I took it. There were several turning points that year—a new marriage with a move to Maryland, and 6 months to get ready for a new position just 15 minutes away from my new home.

An entire chapter could be spent on my Clinical Center experience. The people I met, worked with, and became friendly with were at the leading edge of psychiatric work. Relationships I formed there served me well in later professional experiences. The opportunities to expand my skills in leadership and staff development as well as clinical skills in working with patients and families were without limit. Because we were brand new, I was able to help Gwen develop a staff for each unit, equip the units, set policies, plan educational programs, work with members of other disciplines to establish norms, and get to know everyone who came to look, to stay, or to show new products, films, and treatment strategies (see Part III for one example). We thought we were great and ahead of our time in all dimensions. Indeed, we were in many, and at least trendy in others.

Another opportunity came my way in 1956. I was asked to be a member of the department of psychiatry (led by the renowned Reginald Lourie) at Children's Hospital in Washington, D.C., to serve as psychiatric liaison to the staff in the hospital. We had developed similar roles in nursing at NIH, but I had not worked with all disciplines while there. At Children's, I was to be a participant observer and work with members of all disciplines in a consultative role. It was a terrific job, and again I met outstanding people and formed lasting relationships. I also learned how to develop a grant application that focused on this work. The application was approved and funded, but Sam and I returned to New York, where he did post-master's work in math at Courant Institute, New York University.

That was another turning point for me and a major change in the direction of my career.

ACADEMIA: NYU AND LEHMAN

Until that point I was involved in clinical practice and was quite convinced that it was my destiny. I loved every minute of it, had no interest in formal teaching, and had no desire to pursue a position in education. However, I had come to know many nurse educators during my job at the League, and some of these people had visited the Clinical Center during my time there. One of these people, Dorothy Mereness, was completing her doctorate at Teachers College and planned to take a position at New York University to develop a graduate program there. After her visit to NIH, she wrote to me and invited me to contact her if I ever returned to New York. I did so, and this proved to be another major decision.

It was exciting to be part of a new program and to know that we were at the leading edge of developments in the field. We were the first to focus an entire semester of study on community mental health and on family therapy. Our graduates joined organizations that advanced nursing in these movements. All of the contacts that Dorothy and I had made earlier in our careers were extremely useful as we planned innovative field placements. Martha Rogers was the head of the Division of Nursing at NYU, and she was extremely supportive of Dorothy's efforts.

I was an instructor at NYU from 1956 to 1958 when Sam and I adopted a baby boy, Joshua, and I decided to stay home and devote myself to (almost) full-time motherhood. For the next two years I worked as a mental health consultant at a visiting nurse organization for one day every two weeks and was on call for Dorothy at NYU whenever she needed a fill-in. In 1960 I decided that I was tired of sitting in a Manhattan playground with child caretakers while the mothers were out shopping (not one of my minor vices or pleasures), and that I would get my PhD if I could meet all requirements for a doctoral program. I did qualify, and I completed work for the degree in 1964. In 1963 Sam and I adopted our second child, Charles.

I returned to NYU to plan and direct a new program in child psychiatric nursing. The program was funded by the National Institute of Mental Health, and the first class consisted of six students. Dorothy Mereness left NYU in 1965 to become dean of the school of nursing at the University of Pennsylvania, and I became the director of graduate programs in psychiatric nursing at NYU, a position I held until 1969. When I assumed the position, there were 6 faculty members in my group and we had a total of 22 students in the programs. When I left, there were 13 faculty members and some 42 students in the master's programs. The programs were superb, as was evidenced by the accomplishments of the graduates in later years.

I left NYU to become chair of a new department of nursing at Herbert H. Lehman College, a unit of City University of New York. I had become convinced that the way to really influence the profession was through the professional socialization of students who could deal with the system effectively. The small number of nurses with master's degrees would never be able to achieve the changes that were necessary, and if baccalaureate graduates did not demonstrate differences in their practice from other nurses, I believed that advancement of the profession was in jeopardy.

I knew next to nothing about undergraduate education and set about to study the nursing and health literature and to recruit faculty who could help me in developing a truly innovative undergraduate program. Almost simultaneously, because of my own social interests and because City University had introduced open admissions, I developed a program to recruit and maintain minority students in the new program and to tailor our program for RN transfers.

The baccalaureate program at Lehman was designed to prepare nurses as primary care practitioners. The faculty was committed to this goal, and the program that resulted was cited throughout the nursing and health literature as a model. We were very proud of our accomplishments and of the success of our graduates. Many positions were created for them, and a mark of confidence was the development of new positions within the ambulatory care clinics of the Health and Hospitals Department of the City of New York.

The "team" movement was at its height during this period, and Lehman and Montefiore Hospital, our major affiliate and the instigator of the nursing program, decided to mount other health programs and organize them in the form of a Health Professions Institute. Committees worked on programs in administration, social work, and nursing, and later I became the head of the institute, remaining as chair of the Department of Nursing.

The faculty at Lehman was organized in groups, each with a leader. Decision making was decentralized wherever possible, with strong subgroup and faculty participation in all relevant matters. My style of leadership had become clear to me and to others by this time, and the faculty developed at Lehman was memorable. They were splendid people with extraordinary theoretical and clinical skills, were extremely enthusiastic about what we were doing, and were inspiring to each other and to students. I saw our group as a jewel and we were extremely respected on the Lehman campus and at Montefiore.

So, after seven years, why did I leave my beloved group and my beloved city? The answer is easy. We had accomplished extraordinary things at Lehman for our students and for nursing. Lehman was a liberal arts college without a medical school or hospital of its own. I had concluded that I wanted to test my skills in a larger universe— that of a nursing school in a major university that had a medical school and hospital.

Clearly, the University of Pennsylvania fit the bill. However, I was not too interested in Penn after I received answers to my questions about university support, salaries of faculty, size of the student body, and other vital matters. Barbara Lowery (whom I've come to call the queen of search committees since she always gets her woman), university administrators such as Thomas Langfitt, Vice President for Health Affairs, and Edward Stemmler, dean of the medical school, and a faculty eager for and committed to change were all too persuasive for me to reject.

They were all correct. Penn was right for me, and I was right for Penn. Penn had the combination of factors I was seeking, with so many hurdles for achievement that the challenge for all of us was immense. We had committed to meeting quality goals, and the next few years were full of enormous joint accomplishments. Clearly, the recruitment of faculty and the development of existing faculty within the school were the crucial elements of these accomplishments.

THE UNIVERSITY OF PENNSYLVANIA

The University of Pennsylvania is a multi-racial, multi-ethnic, international learning, teaching, and research community located in a contiguous campus in one of the largest cities in the United States, Philadelphia. It is an urban community of more than 40,000 people, some 22,000 of them students. Penn has many of the structures and problems of any American city of its size. It is the largest private employer in Philadelphia and second only to the City of Philadelphia. The School of Nursing is one of Penn's twelve schools, the smallest of the four undergraduate schools (Arts and Sciences, Engineering, Wharton, Nursing) but larger than all of the graduate schools, with the exception of the School of Medicine.

Penn had the combination of factors I was seeking with so many hurdles for achievement that the challenge for all of us was immense. I and the faculty were committed to meeting quality goals and my years as dean were full of enormous shared accomplishments. Clearly the recruitment of faculty and the development of existing faculty within the school were crucial elements of these accomplishments.

When I came to Penn the School was ready for movement. A core of strong independent thinkers had already developed among the faculty. They were ready for the recruitment of outstanding outsiders, and those who were not ready left the school. With the help of Tom Langfitt, a group of "friends" developed, who eventually became the beginning of our Board of Overseers and who aided in attaining the extraordinary record of private philanthropy we established. Early on we were able to obtain foundation support for a research center and for the development of our primary care programs, both educational and clinical. We accomplished a major goal of integrating faculty practice at the Hospital of the University of Pennsylvania with the establishment of a clinician educator track, analogous to that of the Medical School.

LEAVING THE DEANSHIP AND NEXT STEPS

Normal terms for deans at the University of Pennsylvania are a maximum of twelve years: seven for the first appointment, and after review, five for the second. I stayed beyond that term because we were in the midst of a capital campaign and we knew that another year or so would complete our funding goals. As it turned out, because of the search process, I stayed in the deanship for first one additional year, then two, and finally three, leaving the position in January 1992, fifteen years after I had assumed it. During my tenure as dean, the School had quadrupled in size, built an extraordinary research enterprise, raised a significant amount of money, and achieved recognition as one of the top Schools of Nursing in the United States.

I left the position of dean after accomplishing all of my goals, and because I was very happy at Penn chose to remain with the university despite many possibilities elsewhere. I had, in short, developed a loving and committed relationship to the entire university and was devoted to it and its future in a way that I felt could and should not be duplicated elsewhere. Because there were so many opportunities at Penn for work and colleagueship, I had always said that I could move into the next phase of my career there, and shortly before I left the deanship I started to plan my full time life as a faculty member and "budding researcher." I moved into an endowed chair as Leadership Professor and chose to work on nursing home reform. I was fortunate to find a temporary home at the Institute of Medicine as a Scholar in Residence. The notion of studying the results of OBRA 87 (the Omnibus Budget Reconciliation Act) which had instituted new requirements for nursing homes was suggested to me by Joshua Weiner, a prominent researcher at the Brookings Institution.

I applied first for a small research grant to the Research Foundation at Penn and completed a pilot study which suggested that a fuller survey might offer important findings about what good had come from the new federal requirements. I was fortunate to be funded by the Robert Wood Johnson Foundation to do this work. So in my late 60s I found myself in the most treasured role in all of academia; a funded researcher.

Completing the collection and analysis of data by the end of 1992, I went to the University of California, San Francisco for the winter quarter as a Presidential Chair. I was on leave that semester from my position as Leadership Professor. I started the initial phases of writing the report and later, Sam and I went to France to live briefly in a wonderful house in Provence, working, marketing, cooking, and having a terrific time in our beloved french countryside.

BECOMING INTERIM PRESIDENT

In April of 1993, Sam and I were sitting in a Paris cafe reading the International Herarld Tribune. After months of speculation, there was an item announcing that Sheldon Hackney, President of the University of Pennsylvania, was being nominated for the National Endowment of the Humanities. We returned to Philadelphia a few days later, and on Monday, April 12th, our student newspaper, the *Daily Pennsylvanian* (DP), published a front page article on possible acting presidents. They listed my name way down the page and called me a "long shot." That evening, Barbara Stevens, Vice President and Secretary of Penn, telephoned and asked if I could come to see Al Shoemaker, Chairman of the Board of Trustees, that Thursday. My comment was: "Barbara, if I am a long shot, forget it. I am very tired, just got in from Europe on Saturday and was in Washington today for a meeting. Al doesn't need to make nice to me." Her reply was clear: "Claire, you are no long shot." Sam was less sure of that and comforted by the perception that the University would not ask a former dean of nursing to take this very desired position. "Very desired" are the key words here.

When I met with Al on Thursday, I came prepared to convince him that I was the right person for the job. From the beginning of our interview, it was clear that my "sales" pitch would be unnecessary and that I was being offered the position then and there. Al told me that Sheldon had resigned from the presidency, effective June 30, whether or not his nomination was confirmed. Al also shared with me some information about the people he had talked with about the position and the consensus about his choice of me among a wide variety of faculty, staff, and trustees. It did not take me more than a minute to consider the position, and I walked to the door thinking that I understood the job of president and that I was clear about what needed to be done in an interim period. Al and I had agreed that my propensity for action would not be stymied by my "interimship," and, in fact, was just what he and the other Trustees wanted.

During our meeting, I told Al that I would not be a candidate for the permanent position, but that Sam and I would move into the President's house so that we could be totally immersed in the presidency for the time "we" would hold the position. Sam's willingness to share in this time-limited commitment was a crucial component of my later success.

The following day, Al called and told me that he had decided to change the title from Acting to Interim and that my term would be from July 1, 1993–June 30, 1994. However, he said he would like me to start as soon as possible and take over the formal reins at the Trustee meeting in mid June.

THE FIRST CRUCIAL WEEKS

I accepted the position of Interim President of Penn on April 14, 1993. The next day members of the Black Student League confiscated the student newspaper, the *Daily Pennsylvanian* (DP). "Sides" were taken almost immediately. On the one hand, charges were brought against the students by a faculty member, while on the other, the actions of University police and security guards were severely criticized and subjected to later investigation. The outgoing administration condemned the theft but also talked about the conflict of values that the situation exemplified.

The following week another story with strong racial connotations hit the press, which would become known widely as the "Water Buffalo" incident. It dealt with an event that had occurred in January involving a group of black women students and a white male freshman. Close to midnight on a school night, the women were celebrating the founding of their sorority with traditional chants outside a high rise dormitory. Many students yelled out of the windows, and one student was identified who allegedly called the women "black water buffalos" and told them to go to the zoo if they were looking for a party.

I had dealt with issues of diversity, race relations, and political correctness before, but never at the level of intensity that we were experiencing at Penn. What evolved suddenly was a situation which required all of my clinical knowledge and skills in psychiatric nursing, my administrative and management skills, and my willingness to devote myself—fully and entirely—to healing Penn's internal schisms while moving forward internally and externally to address the many other issues facing the University and its constituents.

I had hoped that between mid April and June 30 it would be possible for Sheldon Hackney and his administration to resolve these two events so that the new team could focus on the healing and resolution of other issues facing the University. This was not possible in either case. What the next weeks revealed was a convoluted system of problem resolution which paralyzed anyone wanting quick action and seemed to penalize accused and accuser. The student judicial system, which had been accepted by all the schools only a few years before, depended heavily on legalistic procedures and maneuvers and left little room for education and mediation. There was little or no oversight of the process of dealing with problems and their resolution.

Two phenomena seemed at work to create this situation. First, all such problems were immediately taken out of the schools and into the central university structure under the Vice Provost for University Life. Thus, deans and faculty were usually unaware of the problems occurring with their students and insulated from the process of resolution. This method, when it worked, was seen to be protective of the academic careers and privacy of the students. However, the method also meant that problems were not handled close to the level at which they occurred and by people who knew the students best.

Second, aside from the specific judicial officers dealing with the students, there did not appear to be accountability built into the hierarchy. If something went wrong, no one seemed responsible or accountable to see that staff were helped and glitches handled. So while some problems were handled very well under this system, others of a more sensitive nature which might have been handled rapidly, fairly, and knowledgeably had the staff flagged their need for help, percolated up to of all places, the President's office. All of the internal and external pressure for a solution was focussed on the President and he was faulted for the mess we were in. Yet the system and policies undergirding it did not include this office in its processes and unless something exploded there was no way the President would normally be informed.

Clearly, in retrospect, both the system and policies were faulty. In addition though, the assumption of academic personnel that reporting lines are meaningless for assumptions of accountability to and for people, was at least as problematic and required attention and change.

Prior to Sheldon's leaving, the two of us met with the young sorority women who had filed the complaint. The meeting was extremely tense, argumentative, and was not successful in reaching a conclusion beneficial to all parties. Still, shortly thereafter, because of what the women perceived as the impossibility of their situation, they decided to withdraw from the case.

The end of judicial procedures did not end the conflict. It merely moved it to new terrains. The press coverage heightened as Sheldon's congressional hearings approached and the "Water Buffalo" issue was covered nationally and internationally. This coverage continued over the summer.

TAKING OVER

When I had originally assessed the positions of President and Provost, I had believed that the Provost was primarily an inside person handling all or most academic matters, relating to students, academic administrators, and faculty, regularly and relatively closely. Given that almost all of the major problems that had hit the press were in that domain it was a surprise to me that the President had been so involved. However, after I took the position and met with staff it became obvious that distances were large between the people handling student issues and the upper levels of the Provost's office. There was no monitoring until a situation had become explosive. Further, the University had become more rigidly bureaucratic in the years that I had not been "noticing" and the infrastructure and superstructure were not functioning flexibly and responsively. Some parts of the President's domain, like Development, were functioning superbly. Others of great importance to the President and the University, particularly at the juncture we were at—i.e. public relations and news—despite excellent staff, had not been able to position Sheldon Hackney in a way to prevent the mess from heightening.

Not only would Sheldon Hackney be leaving at the end of the semester. Almost the entire administration was leaving at the same time. A new Executive VP for Finance had recently been appointed, the Provost and Senior VP for Development and Planning were moving off to presidencies, and an Interim Provost, Marvin Lazerson, Dean of the Graduate School of Education, had been appointed shortly before my appointment. Fortunately, Marv and I had known each other during my deanship and had a good relationship.

Within a week of my accepting the position, Sheldon and I talked about what should be done to put ourselves in a new position for the future. We decided to form a Commission of leaders, internal and external to the university, which would be asked to make recommendations "To promote an academic community in which all members may learn from and be enriched by their similarities and their differences and in which the free exchange of ideas may flourish." I asked the Commission to present a progress report and preliminary recommendations to me and the University Community by January 1994, and present its final report and recommendations by March 31, 1994. These dates would allow me to determine whether or not I would act on their recommendations. My goal was to have as many issues handled during my term in office as possible so that a relatively clean slate would be left for my successor.

During May, meetings were held by the newcomers with the Senior Administrators. The level of anxiety was acute and the style of the meetings seemed to be: Come into the President's office, drop the problems on the meeting table, and leave. The Provost called it the "goose theory of administration." The goslings come around Mother Goose, drop the ____, leave, and she has to clean it up.

I found myself coming home and describing my feelings to Sam as "feeling tears behind my eyes all day." Did I want this job and could I do it? I did what I often do when I am in this kind of funk and what I do with other people in the same sort of totally confounding mood. I reframed the problem. I used my computer in a dialectic process. I started by writing what I was finding and trying to look at it in a new way. In other words, instead of picturing the problem in terms of my own anxiety reaction, I tried to picture it in terms of what others were doing, and what I needed to do to change the picture. So, I wrote some strategies for change and decided to face this head on with the University staff.

At the next meetings I described my style and expectations to my new group. Simply stated: *If you bring in a problem, you'd better bring in one or more solutions. The agenda is mine not yours. We will identify the issues we need to work on and we will establish accountability for those issues.* And that is what we did.

At our first meeting in June, we identified the major "hot button" issues we could expect to face during my presidency. Further, at the June meeting of the Trustees, I committed to a "work list" which would define my term, both in the success of my own work and that of the staff who report to the president. Many items on the work list are ongoing issues at all universities. Others were specific to Penn. In all cases we made substantial progress and several items were achieved completely.

WHY ME?

From the standpoint of the Trustees and Faculty I was an ideal candidate. During my deanship I had travelled far and wide for the School of Nursing and for Penn and was well known among alumni and Trustees. I was well-liked and respected by them, by the Deans, the Faculty, and the new Interim Provost. I had stepped down from a highly successful deanship and thus my accepting the position would not involve a search for a new dean, or an interim appointment in my school. Further, I was clearly not interested in the permanent presidency and would therefore ease the search process.

In 1993 I was just completing a two year term as president of the National League for Nursing and was chairing the Board of Health Promotion and Disease Prevention at the Institute of Medicine. I was frequently called on for consultation by the International Council of Nurses and the World Health Organization, and my work in nursing, health care, psychiatric nursing, and health policy had received wide recognition with posts and honors. I was on one corporate board (Provident Mutual Life Insurance Company) and would be on two others by the next year.

Some years before, the provostship of the University had been open. I was asked to be a candidate for that position and received a great deal of encouragement from the Search Committee. I told the committee and the Trustees who interviewed me that I did not want the job and would reject the opportunity if it was offered to me. But in the process of making a decision about whether or not to pursue it, my husband and I actually made the sort of list of pros and cons that I had heard others talk about, but had never done before. I have often told students, my career unfolded—it was not planned. I had been extremely happy and satisfied in nursing, in nursing administration, and in nursing education as long as the position I held was developing something. The progress in my career came about by evolution when a brief period of boredom would make me ready to seek and accept new challenges.

When I looked at the pros and cons the position of Provost held for me, I realized something. All the parts of the higher administrative position I liked were more likely the parts that would fall under the President. The parts I hated or at least disliked, the more bureaucratic and scheduled, were those that were clearly, at that time anyway, under the Provost. (As stated earlier, this appraisal may have been right then but it was not when I accepted the Interim position.) It was clear that for me at any rate the position of Provost would be a waste since, because of my age (I was already 60), it was unlikely that the job would be a stepping stone to a presidency of a major university. I had a momentary pang that I had not chosen to "distance" myself from a nursing deanship earlier in my career so that I would have had a chance for a presidency like Penn's, but given my general satisfaction with my career the pang was not painful nor prolonged. In fact, when I was asked to consider candidacies elsewhere, there were insufficient enticements to make me leave Penn at that point in my life.

The sequence of events between reading about Sheldon in the International Herald Tribune, reading about me being a "long shot" in the DP, and being offered the position was accompanied by a certainty on my part that this was *my* job and that, of course, unless a strong reason not to take it emerged, I was going to accept immediately. The year or even part of it would be the capstone of my administrative career, and regardless of my success or failure, or my unhappiness or happiness, I would always have it as part of my memories and know I did this job in an institution I cared about.

All this is by way of introducing a retrospective conclusion I have reached about the way I fulfilled the position. As most observers have acknowledged, the accomplishments of the year were beyond anything that can be considered "normal." No letter went unanswered. (Normally, there are about 30 letters received in the president's office daily. During this turbulent time we often received 300 letters.) E-mail and other forms of communication were used extensively. This included closed circuit television for town meetings on campus, talks on campus radio, visits to campus residences, meetings with editorial boards of the major newspapers in Philadelphia, New York, and Washington, and articles in campus journals. We were fortunate to be able to attract the well known debate show "Firing Line" on campus to discuss the issue of free speech. This show, handled by some of the most expert debaters in the country helped to diffuse the issue by putting it in a larger yet discussable context. People felt, and were, in contact. I traveled extensively and visited alumni who had never felt part of the University. We reached new heights in fundraising and in the year raised more money than we ever had in our history. To meet the goals set—and face the new problems which emerged—took more from me and from my husband that anything we had ever experienced. I realized about three quarters of the way through the year that I was approaching the position as though I was a missionary. Because it was a time-limited position, it was possible to continue in this mode, whereas earlier in my career Sam and I would have called a halt to what would have been an impossible and bizarre approach to life. The missionary role is not that foreign to me. I am a nurse and given the problems of the nursing career I had often found myself feeling like a missionary. I had a personal technique for getting myself out of that thinking and unreality and that was to say to myself (as many times as necessary), "Claire, you are not Florence Nightingale, reincarnated." Believe it or not, this self-administered admonition worked and I would snap out of my fugue state and move on with what I could do and still have time for my husband and family.

However, this time was different. My children were grown adults, and my husband was my partner throughout this oddysey—again, always in recognition that it was for one year only!

THE FIRST WOMAN AND A NURSE TO BOOT

Of course it thrilled me to be the first woman chief executive officer of Penn. I knew that the success or failure of my presidency would cast a long shadow on the future but despite the possible outcomes, the appointment sent a message out that Penn was ready for a non-traditional appointment. For this 254 year old University the message for women was hailed with enthusiasm. Hardly less enthusiasm was expressed for the fact that my background, nursing, was even less traditional for such an appointment and the results of that became apparent very quickly. Widely discussed with both seriousness and humor, at Penn and at other universities around the country, was the irony of having a very sophisticated, aggressive medical school dean and health services administrator reporting to a nurse. Both Bill Kelley, the Executive Vice President of the University of Pennsylvania Medical Center and the Dean of the School of Medicine, and I recognized that we needed to confront this issue immediately and I had thought through how I would approach it. Our relationship had always been exceedingly collegial; I had been on the Search Committee which recommended Bill. I told the Board Chairman and Bill that my agenda with him would concern two issues: 1. The fiscal future of the university and 2. Quality of care. Naturally I would still be concerned about the nursing-medicine issues which had often divided us but these would not form the agenda for my presidency (unless I couldn't control myself).

DOES BEING A WOMAN ADMINISTRATOR MAKE A DIFFERENCE?

Many articles have been written over the past few years about the difference between women and men leaders of organizations. A study by the National Foundation for Women Business Owners concluded that "men tend to make quick decisions with limited consultation and put some distance between themselves and their employees. Women, on the other hand, had success with creating a family-like atmosphere at their companies and seeking more outside advice" (Washington Post, July 18, 1994). Other articles have focussed on the more interpersonal strategies women are comfortable with and use, on the reduction in hierarchal methods of administration and management, on the increased focus on communication-listening as well as speaking and sharing information, and on consensus building. These strategies and styles describe much of my own management. While they may be more characteristic of women at large, some women pride themselves on playing so-called "hard ball" in the male model. And I have certainly worked with men who have used similar strategies to those described for women.

Nonetheless, the climate at Penn when I became Interim President called for this interpersonal style with all faculty, deans and other administrators, staff, students, and Trustees. There was a strong sense on the part of the Trustees and the Deans that information was not being shared, that policies were presented when already formed, that problems were not identified before they blew up, and that the separation between "the administration" and others had become severe. Little or no communication occurred proactively with internal or external media and discussion of major issues was too often reactive.

The Interim Provost agreed with me in our goals for Penn and the strategies we used. We both felt strongly that there needed to be broad participation in the issues and real communication about them, which for me as a psychiatric nurse means *real* listening. We also went about identifying and re-identifying the problems and reframing them in ways that might be fresher, clearer and more amenable to solution. We both felt strongly that legal approaches are not immediately substitutable for communication and consensus building in an educational institution, and spent a great deal of time early on and throughout the year building consensus to the greatest degree possible.

THE FAMILY METAPHOR

What cannot be overlooked in my approach to the job was my view of the Penn community as a family. When I became Interim President I called it a dysfunctional family. In a well-functioning family adults do not pull their children into their disputes. In a functional university family there are lots of opportunities for students, faculty, and staff to engage in controversy among themselves and with each other. That is part and parcel of our commitments to freedom of expression and to including all members of our family—faculty, students, and staff—in the discussions of "family matters" that affect their lives and educational attainments. I decided to use many of the techniques of family therapy writ large to address the dysfunctionality I found. Using family metaphors is perhaps more "feminine" than masculine in one's administrative style. There was no question here that the lack of trust needed an immediate fix. A hands-on approach, which might not be important at a different time was vital. The kind of commitment we exemplified early on in the schools, with faculty and staff leaders and with students, began to rebuild the trust that had eroded. Word spread fast in all groups about the meetings we held over the summer and the messages sent via our campus publications kept everyone informed about where we stood on the issues that had divided us.

Some aspects of the woman as administrator and leader were similar to my experiences as a successful nurse. All too often after nurses have performed life-saving or life-improving functions during a patient's hospitalization, the comment made by patient and family is, "the nurses were so nice." Well, the nurse's niceness was lucky for everyone, but it was not niceness that facilitated what appeared to be their effortless acts. What mattered most in the person's hospitalization was that these nice nurses were using knowledge, skill, experience, and smarts in a graceful and smooth way that often prevented their being noticed for what they were.

A November 1994 article in the *Philadelphia Inquirer* about four women leaders at Penn reminded me of this common nursing experience. Personal details were provided about all of us, even in one instance where the subject condemned this approach. Our marriages and children were discussed in detail, some more, some less. In my case there was great emphasis on my warmth and the affection which I inspire.

The paragraph dealing with my accomplishments at Penn went as follows: "She hired a house manager for . . . the president's townhouse on Walnut Street, hung on the ground floor a painting of Ben Franklin womanizing, suspended the speech code, did a 10-city blitz soliciting donations and goodwill from alumni, soothed frayed nerves, and oversaw the drafting of a report on solving Penn's chronic problems."

That was it for my presidency. I could give similar examples from the vignettes about the other three women. After the first positive reaction from readers, the anger from women about trivialization came bursting forth. I had always thought this was a nursing phenomenon but now learned that it was shared with other accomplished women. The more I have thought about this the more I have come to realize that we women do this to each other and don't need men to victimize us in this way. Part of the problem is that each of us is trying to come to terms with the dichotomies, conflicts, and disparate pulls in our lives and we see our own and other's experiences from our own distorted prisms.

What seems to be misunderstood or not understood is how we use our personality attributes within the context of carefully designed strategies for accomplishing goals. The strategies in my case had to do with opening communication internally and externally, building responsibility and accountability, establishing relationships with Penn's wide public, healing the "open" wounds that were apparent and identifying and dealing with more covert problems.

Humanity, warmth, empathy, and other expressionistic characteristics undoubtedly helped and in some cases were essential to the strategies I chose. However, these qualities alone do not do the job. Strategic planning in the deanship and the presidency included setting goals, steps and timetables for their accomplishment and sharing information about their achievement. Some goals were achieved according to the timetable, some delayed, and some preceded our expectations. Nothing was left to chance or hope.

LAST YEARS AT PENN AND BEYOND

When I left the presidency I was welcomed back to the School of Nursing with accolades, fun, and love. The new dean, Dr. Norma Lang, was a major part of making me feel wanted and at home. I was very lucky in this respect as in all others at Penn.

My accomplishments in the deanship and in the presidency were only possible as they reflected a shared commitment with faculty and an understanding on all parts of the importance of strategic planning. As far as the School of Nursing was concerned, faculty members were mutually stimulating, enforced group goals, and supported each other and me. They pushed, pulled, and bolstered each other in varied experiences and reached professional heights I could only have dreamed of in previous experiences.

As I returned to Penn in the Fall of 1994 I began to plan for "early" retirement (my definition of "early" in academia is any time before you're dead). Given that I had some untaken leave, I chose to retire from Penn in June 1996. Sam and I spent some time travelling, sold our beautiful house in Wynnewood, PA, and sublet an apartment in New York City. We wanted to determine whether or not to move back to New York or remain in Philadelphia.

The previous year I had run a conference in Philadelphia as part of the Deans' Distinguished Lecture Series entitled "The Abandonment of the Patient." Working closely with colleagues Dr. Ellen Baer and the journalist Suzanne Gordon, we put together an extraordinary group of health professionals and others who told us their views of what was happening in the for-profit managed care world (see subsequent chapter). I decided that what I wanted to work on in my post-Penn life was the erosion of care of patients and to that end wrote to various Foundations with ideas for study. Dr. Dan Fox of the Milbank Foundation was interested in exploring the subject of the increasing burden of care for nurses and families and I started working with the Foundation before we had a permanent place to live or had made a decision about where to live.

We did decide on New York and my professional life continues to enfold with work with Milbank Memorial Fund, the John A. Hartford Foundation, serving on corporate and not-for-profit boards, speaking, and writing.

What is often missed by people who observe nurses and often, unfortunately by nurses themselves, is the power of the nursing role in the progress of one's career. At every turning point nurses are free to choose to stay in the field in any of the myriad varieties of opportunities available to us or to leave the field for another. This is certainly true at times of educational decisions. Frequently when nurses do move out of nursing but remain in some aspect of the health field, they forget that it is their nursing background that has prepared them for this career change. Whatever I have achieved, the awards I have gotten, the personal rewards I have felt, would not have come my way were I not a nurse. I feel I have given a lot to the profession but I am not even near to repaying what it has given me. I shall always be grateful for the stroke of fortune that brought me to choose this wonderful field.

To be continued . . .

PART ONE

Nursing in the Public Eye: Professional Leadership Issues

Nursing as Metaphor

Claire M. Fagin and Donna Diers

For some time now we have been curious about the reactions of people we meet socially to being told, "I am a nurse." First reactions to this statement include the comment, "I never met a nurse socially before"; stories about the person's latest hospitalization, surgery, or childbearing experiences; the question "How can you bear handling bedpans (vomit, blood)?" or the remark, "I think I need another drink." We believe the statements reflect the fact that nursing evokes disturbing and discomforting images that many educated, middle-class, upwardly mobile Americans find difficult to handle in a social situation. As nurses, we are educated to give comfort, so it is something of a paradox when we make ourselves and others uncomfortable socially.

It is easy to say that some reactions are based on an underlying attitude toward nurses that we tend to think of as a stereotype. But labeling the attitude does not help us explain it or escape it. Perhaps we can deal with the social perception by examining the metaphors that underlie the concept of "nurse"—metaphors that influence not

Note: From the *New England Journal of Medicine*, 309:116–117. (July 14), 1983. It is reprinted here with permission.

only language but also thought and action. An exploration of the metaphorical underpinnings of nursing must start with the etymology of the word "nurse," which is derived from the Latin for "nourish."

Nursing is a metaphor for mothering. Nursing has links with nurturing, caring, comforting, the laying on of hands, and other maternal types of behavior, all of which are seen in our society as essentially mundane and hardly worth noticing. Even the thought of the vertical nurse over the horizontal patient evokes regressed feelings in a woman or man who is told, "I am a nurse." Adults do not like to be reminded, especially in an adult, socially competitive setting, of the child who remains inside all of us.

Nursing is a metaphor for class struggle. Not only does nursing represent women's struggles for equality, but its position in the health world is that of the classic underdog, struggling to be heard, approved, and recognized. Nurses constitute the largest occupational group in the health-care system (2.6 million). They work predominantly in settings that are dominated by physicians and in which physicians represent the upper and controlling class. Dominant groups yield ground reluctantly, especially to those who are regarded as having simply settled for a job instead of choosing a more prestigious profession.

Nursing is a metaphor for equality. Little social distance separates the nurse from the patient or the patient from other patients in the nursing-care setting, no matter what the social class of each. Nurses themselves make little distinction in rank among persons with widely varying amounts of education. Nurses are perceived as members of the working class, and although this perception is valuable to the patient when he or she is ill and wants to be comforted, it may be awkward to encounter one's nurses at a black-tie reception, where working-class people do not belong.

Among physicians, nursing may be a metaphor for conscience. Nurses see all that happens in the name of health care—the neglect as well as the cures, the reasons for failure as well as those for success. The anxiety, not to mention the guilt, engendered by what nurses may know can be considerable. Nurses recognize that many of the physician's attempts to conquer death do not work. They are an uncomfortable reminder of fallibility.

Nursing is a metaphor for intimacy. Nurses are involved in the most private aspects of people's lives, and they cannot hide behind technology or a veil of omniscience as other practitioners or technicians in hospitals may do. Nurses do for others publicly what healthy persons do for themselves behind closed doors. Nurses, as trusted peers, are there to hear secrets, especially the ones born of vulnerability. Nurses are treasured when these interchanges are successful, but most often people do not wish to remember their vulnerability or loss of control, and nurses are indelibly identified with those terribly personal times.

Thanks to the worst of this kind of thinking, nursing is a metaphor for sex. Having seen and touched the bodies of strangers, nurses are perceived as willing and able sexual partners. Knowing and experienced, they unlike prostitutes are thought to be safe—a quality suggested by the cleanliness of their white uniforms and their professional aplomb.

Something like the sum of these images makes up the psychological milieu in which nurses live and work. Little wonder, then, that some of us have been badgered (at least in our earlier days) about our choice of career. Little wonder, then, that nurses have had to develop a resilience required of few other professionals. Little wonder, too, that it is so difficult for us to reply to our detractors. One may wonder why any self-respecting, reasonably intellectual man or woman chooses nursing as a lifelong career. Our students at Pennsylvania and Yale are regularly asked questions like this by family, friends, and acquaintances: "Why on earth are you becoming a nurse? You have the brains to be a (doctor, lawyer, other)." All of them, long before entering schools such as ours, must answer this question for themselves and their questioners in a way that permits them to begin and to continue nursing. Their responses and ours frequently focus on the role of the nurse, the variety and mobility possible in a nursing career, or the changing nature of the profession. That kind of answer doesn't get to the heart of the problem in the mind of the questioner. Although it may elicit an "Oh, I didn't realize that," it doesn't make any permanent points for anyone. The right answer has to address the metaphors, since these are the reasons for the concern. The answer must convey the feeling of satisfaction derived from the caring role; indifference to power for its own sake; the recognition that one is a doer who enjoys doing for and with others; but most of all, the pleasure associated with helping others from the position of a peer rather than from the assumed superordinate position of some other professions.

The metaphors, if we turn them around, can easily work to explain our position. Intimacy—why shrink from the word, even while we educate our listeners about its finer meaning—equality, conscience, and the many qualities of motherhood (another word that can usefully be separated from its stereotype) are exactly what draw people into nursing and keep them there.

If we could manage to be wistfully amused by the reactions we evoke at social events rather than defensive, life would be easier. Educated, middle-class, upwardly mobile—we are indeed the peers of others at these social gatherings. We are peers informed about disease prevention, the promotion of health, and rehabilitation. We are not disinterested experts but advocates, even for those who misinterpret us. Others may be only dimly aware of our role, but it is rooted deep in our history and exemplified by the great nursing leaders who have moved society forward: Lavinia Dock, so active in pursuing women's rights; Lillian Wald (a nurse whom society has preferred to disguise as a social worker), who developed the Henry Street Settlement and educated all of us in understanding and approaching health and social problems; Margaret Sanger, who faced disdain, ignominy, and imprisonment in her struggle to educate the public about birth control; and Sister Kenny, who was once the only hope for polio victims.

So much for the metaphors of others. For ourselves? We think of ourselves as Florence Nightingale—tough, canny, powerful, autonomous, and heroic.

CHAPTER THREE

Nursing Comes of Age

Joan E. Lynaugh and Claire M. Fagin

W e wish to celebrate a strange and paradoxical subculture in American society: a group whose conflicts internally and externally have been well recorded; a group that confronts barriers to advancement and even survival—barriers that stem from deep social, economic, and professional ambivalences about its responsibilities and its privileges.

This essay is grounded in two historic realities: first, nursing is made up of individuals from heterogeneous class, ethnic, and racial backgrounds; and, second, the mission of nursing, giving care, is undervalued in our society. These two realities fuel contemporary debate and underlie the questions that we argue every day. Is nursing a profession or simply a skilled occupation? Does it matter? Should nursing continue to try to collaborate with medicine, or should we focus on competition? Can we succeed in attending new nurses if we cling to our caregiving, altruistic mission? How does oppression of nurses as women fit into this story? Why is nursing reaffirmed as being crucial to society only in times of shortage and systematically devalued at all other times?

Note: This is an updated version of an article published in *IMAGE: Journal of Nursing Scholarship*, Vol. 20, No. 4, Winter 1988. It is reprinted here with permission.

This confluence of paradoxes, problems, and characteristics of nursing development and its current situation can be responded to in two ways. One is to bewail our failures and accept their inevitability in the face of a historically hostile environment. The other is to wonder at and celebrate the extraordinary accomplishments of nurses, mostly of the wrong sex and social class, who have the wrong history and education, who persist and achieve in spite of being held back by some of the most powerful forces in our society.

The perspective of celebration is vital. It would be supremely ironic if nursing and its public were to fail to recognize our victories. If we do not understand accurately where we are now, we will continue to fight the battles of yesterday and squander the resources that we need for addressing the problems of today and tomorrow. In this chapter, we draw from the past and the present to propose a way of positioning nursing for the twenty-first century.

We identify some paradoxes of the nursing profession—enduring dilemmas—characteristics of our work that are, for nursing, both panacea and poison. We explore five fundamental and overarching descriptors and predictors of nursing's situation: nursing's mission—caregiving, nursing's fit with the economic system, gender—the women's issue, oppression, and our preoccupation with professional status.

A SOCIETY THAT SYSTEMATICALLY UNDERVALUES CARE

The assumption in our culture is that nurses substitute for family members and servants. For 100 years, during those times when self-care and family care no longer suffice, we have experimented with ways to transfer the job of "caring for another" from the family to nursing. We cast our work in educational, assistive, empathetic, sustaining, and managerial terms. We say that we "put the patient in the best condition for nature to act on him (Nightingale 1860/ 1969) or that we "assist the individual . . . in . . . those activities . . . that he would perform unaided if he had the necessary strength, will or knowledge" (Henderson, 1966, p. 15). When nursing was invented (i.e., when women of the nineteenth century conceptualized how the substitutive function of nursing should be carried out), nursing was seen as assuring a safe environment, sharing moral and scientific knowledge, and sustaining the whole person.

The idea that each specific disease should have a specific cure did not really take over until the end of the nineteenth century. Nursing, of course, was invented well before that—in the 1860s and 1870s. It was intended for American nursing to deal with the individual and collective problems created by dependence in the circumstance of illness. And, it is important to stress, the way nurses conceived of illness at that time was representative of the society at large; that is, although the sick hoped to be cured by medicine, they only hoped to be cured, they did not really expect it, the way we now expect a cure. Most individuals believed that health and illness depended on a balance between one's personal, inherited constitution, and the surrounding environment. Nurses supported personal resistance to the ravages of disease and controlled the environment.

At first, most patients were persons who did not have family caregivers because they were poor and isolated through immigration or destruction of the family, or because they were a danger to their families as a result of contagion or insanity. By the end of the nineteenth century, however, more and more Americans were delegating their own care to nurses rather than to family members because they thought it was safer or more convenient and because they could afford it.

Just when the success of nursing as a substitute for family caregiving began to be realized, things began to change dramatically in health care. By the beginning of the twentieth century, an interventionist, specific disease model of medicine began to dominate. This model replaced older, more conservative, nineteenth century "watchful waiting" approaches to sickness. With the success of the germ theory in explaining infectious illness, "disease" came to be the moral and logical organizing device for the payment for care. In the twentieth century encounters between health care providers and patients were justified by the existence of real or presumed disease (Rosenberg, 1987). As Rosenberg pointed out, "Specialization exemplified and exacerbated a more general tendency of medicine toward the reductionist and technological; its existence helped justify and act out the powerful image of the hospital as scientific institution" (pp. 174–175).

By 1900 the dilemma of how to constitute nursing's task of substitute caregiving in the face of these sweeping changes was confronted in hospitals most of all. In addition to the socially mandated task of substituting for the family, nurses were asked to assume the institutionally mandated task of substituting for the physician. The myriad tasks associated with diagnosis and therapy began to dominate the interior life of hospitals and the work day of nurses. Nurses, like other Americans, were captivated by the successes that disease-specific models of care seemed to achieve over the frightening toll caused by epidemic illness. For the first 60 or 70 years of the twentieth century, nursing essentially "tagged along" with this change in the way that health care was defined and delivered. Moreover, hospital nurses made possible many of the surgical and medical interventions that came to characterize care of the sick.

Now, at the start of the twenty-first century, these acute care, interventionist models and disease-focused designs for payment for care seem to have become a problem. They fail to correspond in a functional way with our increasingly perceived need for providing care for children, the old, the chronically ill, and the dying. There is heightening concern that these needs are in competition with each other for declining resources. We Americans believe that we have the best health care in the world but we are unhappy and worried about the cost of the care as well as the number of people not receiving care, and we are uneasy about our individual prospects with respect to long-term and chronic care (Pokorny, 1988).

These concerns fit superbly with nursing's caregiving mission. Throughout its 80 years of collaboration with the acute care interventionist model, nursing has held on to its ideology of holism and family-based care. Let us celebrate what nurses have done to build that which is best about hospitals—caregiving, safety, competence, and continuity where these ingredients are possible. Nursing continues to espouse the idea that illness affects persons and families, that care should be organized around individuals and families rather than diseases.

Person-based care has been practiced by nurses working in visiting nurse societies, in nursing homes, and in private duty as well as in multiple other arenas of practice. Nursing has insisted on defining itself as the profession that assists ill persons without regard for their cure potential.

Recall that our discipline grew out of a public demand for knowledgeable caregivers. Nursing is a response to the insistence by modern society that dependent members not be abandoned to their fate and, beyond that, that the sick require informed and reliable care. We should celebrate the roles that nursing plays in ameliorating the harsher aspects of a highly individualistic, productivity-oriented society, the ideology of holism, adaptation favoring survival, reform rather than passive acceptance, and altruism rather than the self-serving exploitation of others.

But we should also analyze critically our decisions about how those caregiving resources are used and to whose benefit they are applied. We need to be sure that nursing resources are applied first to the public good; vital nursing services should not be diverted to preserve institutions or support other professional groups.

NURSING AND THE ECONOMIC SYSTEM

Nursing has its origins in unpaid domestic work and powerful historic links with religiously inspired human services. Neither domestic service nor the religious sisterhoods are the route to individual financial success. Paradoxically, nursing also served as one of the most successful routes to respectable paid work for women. This is a complicated story; we will explore part of it.

Except for care of the insane and the infectious, the military and the very poor there was minimal government involvement or investment in the care of the sick until after World War II. Nursing developed in the private sector, which, in the nineteenth century, attracted little public debate. What the private sector developed in the way of health care services was pretty much what the dominant middle class thought was important. Community leaders, businessmen, and philanthropists wanted to buy, both for themselves and for those whom they thought worthy of their charity, those services that they thought counted for biological survival and freedom from pain or dysfunction.

It is important to remember that not much money circulated in the health care system before World War II. Neither hospitals nor physicians nor medical researchers, and certainly not nurses, resembled those of today, either in affluence or influence. For hospitals, a crucial crutch was the minimally paid pupil nurse. They subsidized American hospitals and made it possible for a labor-intensive business to survive and even grow in a cash-starved sector of the economy.

The pupil nurses were willing to trade their time, labor, and sometimes their health for the title "graduate nurse" because nursing constituted paid work for women—and this was respected by society. The private duty practice that most of these graduate nurses entered offered an avenue to self-support, however unstable. By the 1920s there were nearly 2,000 training schools churning out graduates into the private duty market. Most of these nurses worked in their patients' homes. Ironically, if the patients stayed home and paid the private duty nurse to care for them, they did not use the hospital. Thus the graduates of the hospital training school were in competition with their alma maters for paying patients (Reverby, 1983).

The patients were increasingly willing and able to pay for health care services. It is important not to lose sight of the attractiveness and significance to the American public of nursing care. Our predecessors had pride and confidence in their product. As individual practitioners, however, they experienced great difficulty in competing successfully with institutions. A second irony in this private duty-hospital competition is that the hospitals were led most often by other nurses. Christopher Parnell, the medical superintendent at University Hospital in Ann Arbor, explained in 1920 that hospital administration frequently attracted physicians who were "medical derelicts," whereas "the reasons for the almost universal employment of trained nurses as hospital executives has been simply that a higher quality of intelligence could be purchased for the money than could be secured in the service of men in the positions" (Parnell, 1920).

A third element of this strange story is the unknown cost of nursing care. Except for private duty, nurses have been paid salaries by institutions that in turn sell their services either by renting beds by the day or selling nursing visits one at a time. Hospital-based nursing care was rarely singled out either as an expense or as a source of revenue. So, except for the earliest nurse-run hospitals, no one, including the nurse supervisor and the hospital administrator, kept track of the real cost of nursing although it was the central service that the institution provided.

Perhaps because students were the laborers and because most hospitals were either benevolent institutions or tax supported, no "outsiders" demanded an accounting. Thus hospitals could and did operate under exceptionally simple and uninformative budgets. The outcome, however, was to hide the real costs of nursing care until the 1950s. Then, when student labor began to be withdrawn from the hospitals by the reformation or closing of diploma schools, pained outcries were heard. As long as retrospective reimbursement from insurers closed the gap, however, we still did not confront the real costs of nursing care. The distress over the cost of health care has made us begin to consider seriously accounting the actual cost and revenue of hospital nursing care; this belated concern was accelerated in 1983 by the prospective payment system.

During the 1950s, nurses also began to insist on improving their economic situation and turned to the tried and true methods of collective bargaining. Other workers in American society had organized much earlier, but for a long time nurses, isolated and altruistic, did not move. They tended to accept the economic facts of life as they were. Shirley Titus (1952), one of the founders of the movement to improve the economic plight of nurses, summed it up in 1952:

> As I have given thought to the situation, it has seemed to me that the nurse within the four walls of her job—and her job has practically constituted her whole waking life—has been like a sleeper who has slept serenely on while a great battle—a battle for human freedom and the rights of the common man—was being waged. But eventually the sleeper awakens. (pp. 1109–1110)

The sleeper is now *almost* fully awake. We are learning to price our services in a way that is equitable both to the consumer and to the provider. We have learned that altruism and subsidization have too high a price; they devalue our work, they impair recruitment, and they burden unfairly a vital social service.

We have not touched directly on the impact of technology on the economic status of nursing. Nor have we brought public health and visiting nursing into the economic story. We will leave this question of economic fit by making only two points. First, nursing is a product that Americans have proved again and again that they want to buy. Second, Americans have no easy way of knowing what our services are worth or should cost. The reasons for this odd state of affairs rest in the hidden, intimate nature of nursing, in its altruistic and domestic origins, and most of all in the great cultural reluctance to admit to the real costs of the nursing services we seem to want.

The creativity in hiding these costs is astonishing (Lynaugh, 1987). American ingenuity figured out how to use pupils instead of trained nurses to care for patients and created turnover (which we used to think was good) by refusing to employ married nurses. We kept salaries down by labeling women's wages "supplemental." We allowed hospitals to fix wages. We excluded nurses from direct insurance-based reimbursement. We argued that we could not afford to acknowledge the concept of comparable worth (Feldberg, 1984).

Nursing has an essential product; and our public is beginning to acknowledge this reality with economic rewards instead of kind testimonials. With help from consumers we chip away at restrictions on third-party reimbursement. We are out from under the yoke of hospital domination of our educational system. Demand for our services drives entry-level salaries up even in these cost-conscious times, particularly when the spectre of shortage looms. Nurse-midwives, nurse practitioners, psychiatric clinical specialists, nurse anesthetists, neonatal nurses, and gerontology nurses prove their worth directly, and the purchasing public responds.

Upwards of 20,000 nurses have started independent business ventures. Nurses in most states are allowed to bill private insurers directly for their services and have prescription privileges. Medicare restrictions for reimbursement for nurse practitioners and advanced practice nurses have been removed. All of these accomplishments have been in the face of strong, organized opposition.

All of these efforts were strengthened by the report of the Office of Technology Assessment (1986), which found that nurse practitioners were not being used to their fullest potential. The study concluded that, if their services were covered, access to care would be improved for underserved populations, and cost savings could be achieved. Currently, efforts are being made to find acceptable cost accounting systems for hospital nursing services, and several models have been developed and are being tested. We are documenting nursing interventions and costs so as to provide the data necessary for third-party reimbursement for nursing care in any setting (Fagin, 1986).

These economic accomplishments have been in the face of strong, organized opposition from the American Medical Association and, early on, from the insurance industry. Recently the insurance industry has changed its position, having recognized the possible cost savings of alternate health care providers, specifically nurses.

GENDER—THE WOMEN'S ISSUE

The history of nursing shows that women are dominated by the male values of American society and deterred from their goals by implicit and explicit acceptance of those values by the masses. Today 95.1% of Registered Nurses are women; while there have been, and continue to be, men in the profession who are major contributors, nursing's female image has deterred men from entering nursing in the numbers necessary to change its femaleness. How can nursing succeed unless we become a woman-valued work group? We have struggled with domination by male physicians, administrators, and board members for almost all of our 100-year history. We have tried isolation, accommodation, isolation again, collaboration, demands for equality, and negotiation. A woman's occupation with superb women leaders, yet dominated by men from other disciplines, is a paradox that is tied to the economic dilemma but its complexity goes beyond economic equity.

Lavinia Dock lived and practiced across both centuries of our existence. She was an author, feminist, and pacifist. Of all of the turn-of-the-century leaders, she probably understood best the American culture. She said it simply: "The status of nursing . . . depends on the status of women" (Dock & Stewart, 1920, p. 338). Nursing is a woman's profession because it is nursing.

There is another irony: Americans have an agenda of self-actualization and productivity. The vital role of nursing in relation to American social priorities has led to reluctance on the part of the public to come to grips with the worth of nursing, that is, to acknowledge how much it really costs to buy the freedom that nursing offers American families. As long as women were willing to subsidize the development of hospitals, high-technology care, and care of the poor through their own low wages, America was free to expand these services at relatively low cost.

Nursing was born in the first women's movement in the midnineteenth century, bred in the second movement during the drive for the vote, and reached a startling political and professional maturity in the last years of the twentieth century. The renaissance of nurse-midwifery and the nurse practitioner movements can be seen as illustrations of nursing's sending out "pseudopods" of services desired by the public but left unattended through restrictions created by both medicine and nursing. These movements achieved the bringing together of nurses and consumers of nursing care. Nurse-midwives and nurse practitioners confronted the interdependence of medicine and nursing, which had been hidden by medical dominance. This was a painful and difficult process since it involved giving up the more comfortable strategy of isolation from medicine adopted by nursing in the 1950s and 1960s. In this new interdependence, the qualities that nurses value were allowed to influence overtly the interaction. Supportiveness, compassion, concern for others, concern for human relationships are qualities seen by some feminists as being essentially self-sacrificing (Blum, Homiak, Housman, & Shaman, 1976). Nurses retained and continue to display these qualities despite value shifts that define "good" women's behaviors as those valued by men.

A critical mass of women leaders is found in all countries including those in the Third World—nurses working in practice and education as well as in associated health field roles in governments throughout the world. Reports at meetings of the International Council of Nurses—give superb evidence of social reform and leadership in which all women could take pride and satisfaction. Hundreds of stories are told at these meetings of nurses' taking leading roles in providing services to the unemployed, to people with AIDS, and to other populations at risk. Nurses are at the front lines of care and the administration of health care in its vast variety of settings throughout the world. Many can now also be found in both the corporate world and law in positions that were anticipated by the "upward and onward" clichés in their high school year books.

The first case on comparable worth was brought by a group of nurses in Denver, Colorado, and one of the first suits brought by women faculty members seeking comparable salaries occurred at the University of Washington, stimulated by the faculty in the School of Nursing. The ANA served as amicus curiae in that case. In the late 1980s, in Illinois a case is being brought and a Pennsylvania suit was won (Holcomb, 1988). But, we still have trouble behaving like winners; and we are some distance away from consensus on Melosh's

(1982) call for a "generous and inclusive program [leading] toward expanded authority for all nurses" (p. 210).

OPPRESSION

One explanation for fragmented group behavior may rest in the concept of oppression. Roberts (1983) argues that nursing can be considered an oppressed group because it has been controlled by forces outside itself that "had greater prestige, power, and status and that exploited the less powerful group" (pp. 21–22). Oppressed groups commonly feel self-hatred and low self-esteem.

Nurses are being targeted for a new public relations effort because it is apparent that we are caught up in self-flagellating and group-flagellating behavior—the oppressors' "blame the victim." Oppressed individuals are given to intragroup conflict, and this is often used by the oppressors to illustrate that the group cannot come together, cannot govern themselves, cannot organize. Examples of these two characteristics are found in the constant accusations that we are unable to speak with one voice. Our intragroup conflict is evident in any discussion about levels in nursing education.

To remain oppressed, groups must be kept in their place. Only by behaviors that keep nurses "down" can the other players stay "up" (Myrdal, 1944). Nurses are ambivalent about protesting real or perceived threats and generally prefer accommodation. But nursing needs to examine the ends served by accommodation versus planning a coherent, strategic form of protest to conditions that, at the very least, threaten the performance of nursing. Individuals who protest may accomplish some important goals. One is to demonstrate that protest does not hurt and may even advance the protester. Group protest, of course, is much safer and certainly more potent, but so far it has been used insufficiently in nursing. Perhaps this is because, as Reverby (1987) suggests, "Occupational loyalty, the basic consciousness necessary to begin a professionalizing and standardizing effort, [is] difficult to elicit within nursing" (p. 122). Of the five discussed here, this dilemma is the most difficult to celebrate since the *un*oppressed, though numerous, are far less representative than we would like of the group as a whole.

PROFESSION VERSUS OCCUPATION

All groups with special social functions (i.e., professions) are defined both by their social relevance and by their value orientations rather than by any empirical fact. Although the work of nursing continued to be important fundamentally, in the early part of the twentieth century something that presumably was better (i.e., cure and prevention of disease) was being offered. Our rhetoric remained unrelentingly holistic; it included the individual, the family, and the environment and romanticized the view of the nurse as advocate for patients and their care during those times when the patients (clients) are unable to do those things for themselves. Retaining a holistic and romantic concept while seeking professional status through the university is yet another example of nursing's survival in a climate oppressive and antagonistic to both its basic essence and its belief system.

It seems strange that few among us are willing to relinquish the term "professional" from our identity—"strange" because it is irrational to consider that all registered nurses are professional no matter what their preparation. If we do, there does not seem to be much meaning to the term. If we could get the term "professional" out of our language we might be better able to stratify and segment our group. Melosh (1982) believes that, "as a strategy for nursing, professionalization is doomed to fail; as an ideology, professionalism divides nurses and weds its proponents to limited and ultimately self-defeating values" (p. 16). In addition to the resistance to change created by moral and religious overtones and undertones, professionalization draws boundaries that may be resisted strongly by members of the group who are seen as outside those boundaries. When they are the clear majority, this opposition undercuts and often makes futile efforts to "upgrade," achieve power and achieve autonomy and other essentials of professionalization.

Early public health nurses came closer than any other nurses to claiming the privileges of professionals. Their work was relatively unconfined, they were independent and they had an esprit de corps and a special identity. They did not make common cause with other nurses because they relished their own autonomy and their special relationship with philanthropic supporters (Buhler-Wilkerson, 1983). Later, when medicine challenged and succeeded in aborting this movement, their lack of common cause with the masses of nurses brought little support during the years of their demise. An interesting and contrasting case in point is the experience of nursing and nurse-midwifery. For decades the nurse-midwife group was shunned by nurses, and the feeling was mutual. For more than a decade now this noxious and ultimately destructive situation has changed dramatically. Nurse-midwives are very much a part of nursing and its leadership and support and are supported by other nurses in their quest for independence, autonomy, power, and access to the reimbursement stream. Yet nurse-midwives are facing new pressures both within and outside of their group as their own fragile professionalism is just being achieved. Their problems mirror the larger questions of power, control, occupational loyalty, and group cohesion.

Achieving professionalism for a caring discipline with a holistic philosophy, predominantly female and oppressed, with limited access to the funding stream may be a laughable objective. But celebrate what we have accomplished.

Most national nursing organizations have endorsed the baccalaureate degree as the minimum entry-level credential for professional nursing. The public has told us in poll after poll that they "believe" nurses are educated at least at the four year college level. They have also told us of their trust in nurses. In the episodic shortage and oversupply cycles the demand for baccalaureate educated nurses has not flagged and the need for nurses with higher degrees is expected to increase. A serious shortage of faculty is already being felt and the aging of the nursing workforce presages a new crisis.

The acceptance of nurse practitioners and advanced practice nurses is one of the hallmarks of nursing coming of age. Nurses appear to be the providers of choice in case manager roles. The data show that nursing affects patient outcomes and contributes to the goals of a competitive health care system (OTA, 1986). Convincing evidence for hospitals' and physicians' support of professional status are such studies as the one completed at George Washington University, which compared the outcome (mortality) of 5,020 patients in intensive care at 13 hospitals. In intensive care units that had the lowest mortality, nurses operated with a high degree of autonomy, were the best educated and had independent responsibilities (Knaus, Draper, Wagner, & Zimmerman, 1986).

Several foundations have been instrumental in enhancing the professionalism of nursing. A major initiative was the Robert Wood Johnson Foundation Teaching Nursing Home Project. This program proposed to improve the quality of care provided in nursing homes through linkage of selected nursing homes to university schools of nursing. It was also intended that nursing students might be attracted to long-term care as an attractive career opportunity because of the role modeling of expert clinicians. Now completed, the project is being evaluated and by all accounts appears to have been successful in improving the quality of care in the nursing homes involved and increasing the professional status of the carers (Aiken, Mezey, Lynaugh, & Buck, 1985; Joel, 1986; Mezey, Lynaugh, & Cartier, 1988).

The most important reason to celebrate achievements in nurse professionalism are the extraordinary accomplishments of nurse researchers in conducting research that focuses on patient care and systems improvement. The frequently cited study of Brooten (1986) is a case in point. Brooten et al. studied the effects of early discharge of low birth weight infants when the family was supported by a perinatal nurse clinician according to a specific regimen. The results were positive for the families, and the cost benefits were significant. Publication in the *New England Journal of Medicine* brought a great deal of attention to the team and to the nursing profession, and, like the study on intensive care, cited above, provided additional credibility for the effectiveness of the credentialed nurse specialist.

As nursing comes of age no achievement seems as paradoxical as the establishment of the National Institute for Nursing Research, which recognizes and supports the professional status of nursing at the uppermost level, while the occupational membership refuses to come to terms with preparation for such status at the entry level.

MOVING TO COMING OF AGE

Biologist and philosopher Rene Dubos made clear that biological success in all its manifestations is fundamentally a measure of fitness (and he meant fitness to survive); fitness requires never-ending efforts of adaptation to the environment, which is ever changing (Dubos, 1959). So, we will try to develop a picture of the environment and the fitness of nursing now and in the coming decades—an epidemiologic picture.

According to Olshansky and Ault (1986), epidemiologic scholars outline a four-state historical sequence of events, beginning with the age of pestilence and famine, when infectious diseases such as infant diarrhea, tuberculosis, and small pox killed children and young adults frequently and at young ages. This was followed by the age of receding pandemics—an era of falling death rates from infectious illnesses, probably resulting from rapid improvement in sanitation and nutrition in the nineteenth century and creating a redistribution of death from the young to the old. Midway into the twentieth century we reached a plateau—the age of degenerative and man-made diseases, when the major causes of death were heart disease, cancer, and stroke; life expectancy reached into the seventies. Now, a rapid decline in mortality signals a new era—the age of "delayed degenerative diseases." Nursing's current and future priorities must reflect this epidemiologic reality.

Although it is important that we continue our concern about the care, treatment, and prevention of acute illnesses, our experience teaches us that acute infectious illnesses do not very often kill our children. Lack of prenatal care and violence do. Our parents no longer succumb early to acute pneumonia, the "old man's friend," but recover to face an uncertain future and need help with everyday living. A nation that places all of its resources in cure-oriented diagnosis and treatment of disease shortchanges the growing part of the population who require care and support. All health care providers must explore and adapt their educational and service structures to meet the needs of the current era. Nursing, the most adaptable of all of the providers, conceives its future and chooses among socially and ethically sound alternatives to accommodate to this "age of delayed degenerative diseases."

CONCLUSIONS

We have explored five enduring dilemmas or paradoxes affecting nursing since its origin in this country. In each instance we illustrated, if not pure "panacea," at least extraordinary accomplishments yielding more than enough reason to celebrate where we are in 2000 and giving us confidence to plan for the future.

The entire health care system has been built on the backs of nurses—first on the training-apprentice model of free service, then on the poorly paid masses of service-oriented, educated, but mainly female workers. We can celebrate thousands of nurses and leaders at multiple levels. There are hundreds of experiments in innovative models of nursing practice, which address the structural problems that diminish the participation and effectiveness of nursing; these are new examples of managed care and differentiated practice and creatively responsive services for the elderly in nursing homes and in the community. Nurse entrepreneurs are at the leading edge of market developments in health care. Nurse researchers are exploring issues ranging across the entire spectrum of patient care as well as the social and biological sciences. In many cases this research has significant cost implications. Nurses are in distinguished, elected and appointed positions nationally and regionally, and nurse lobbyists are considered to be among the most effective in Washington.

Many nurses are "at the table" of decision making at local and national levels in governmental and private groups that customarily are closed to women. We believe that this shows that nurses have much greater access to power than we recognize. The concern that many men express about possible conspiratorial behavior when women collect is an indicator of the potential power of women and nurses to foster change. Clearly it is one reason for the continued opposition of the AMA and the AHA to upgrading nursing education for the masses. After all, with more education, we might have even more articulate movers and shakers and be even more dangerous to the status quo.

Coming of age requires that we look beyond the splendid minority in our group and recognize that within our unrecognized and invisible majority are many extraordinary contributors to the lives of individuals who must be brought into visibility within the profession and to the public. The accomplishments of our leaders have meaning only when they support, sustain, make sense of, and forward the work of those for whom the leaders speak and act.

In clarifying the persistent and pervasive paradoxes of the profession we must ask how we have accomplished so much in the century of our existence. We believe that it is the common link to caring that brings nurses together. It is the link that brought us all to this great field of oppression and opportunity; it is this which keeps us persisting despite the seduction of less problematic fields or work.

It doesn't take a horticulturist to know that a beautiful tree has a very limited life span when the roots are unattended. It is crucial to include all nurses in our pursuit of autonomy, authority, and development. Our leading thinkers must collaborate in solving the problems of the two thirds of nurses who work in hospitals. We need new organizations of work to enhance the position of all nurses and patients in the special modern institutions created for care of one group through reliance on the other. Together we can ensure that there is enfranchisement and expanded authority for all nurses while we struggle to agree to a different and more unified future. We can learn from each other, build our broad base for action through mutual respect, recognize and cherish our diversity, and come of age as a profession by using to its fullest our unusual combination of caring, ambition, initiative, smarts, and true grit.

REFERENCES

Aiken, L., Mezey, M., Lynaugh, J., & Buck, C. (1985). Teaching nursing homes. *American Geriatrics Society, 33,* 196–201.

American Hospital Association (1988). *Survey of hospitals.* Chicago: AHA.

Blum, L., Homiak, M., Housman, J., & Shaman, N. (1976). Altruism and women's oppression. In C. Gould & M. Wartofsky (Eds.), *Women and philosophy.* New York: Putnam.

Brooten, D., Kumar, S., Brown, L., Butts, P., Finkler, S., Bakewell-Sachs, Gibbons, A., & Delivoria-Papadoponlus, M. (1986). A Randomized Clinical Trial of Early Hospital Discharge and Home Follow-Up of Very-Low-Birth-Weight Infants. *New England Journal of Medicine, 315,* 934—939.

Buhler-Wilkerson, K. (1983). False dawn: The rise and decline of public health nursing in America, 1900–1930. In E. C. Lagemann (Ed.), *Nursing history, new perspectives, new possibilities* (pp. 89–106). New York: Teachers College Press.

Dock, L., & Stewart, I. (1920). *A short history of nursing.* New York: Putnam.

Dubos, R. (1959). *Mirage of Health.* New York: Harper and Row.

Fagin, C. (1986). Opening the door on nursing's cost advantage. *Nursing and Health Care, 7,* 356–358.

Feldberg, R. (1984). Comparable worth: Toward theory and practice in the United States. *Signs: Journal of Women, Culture and Society, 10,* 311–328.

Henderson, V. (1966). *The nature of nursing: A definition and its implications for practice, research and education.* New York: Macmillan.

Holcombe, B. (1988, June). *Ms Magazine,* 78.

Joel, L. (1986, November 14). *Comparison of clinical outcomes.* Paper presented to the conference, Teaching Nursing Home Program: a Perspective on Education/Service Collaboration, Rutgers College of Nursing, Newark, NJ.

Knaus, W. A., Draper, E., Wagner, D., & Zimmerman, J. (1986). An evaluation of outcome from intensive care in major medical centers. *Annals of Internal Medicine, 104,* 410–418.

Lynaugh, J. (1987, June 9). Riding the yo-yo: The Work and Worth of Nursing in the 20th Century. Paper presented to the conference, Nurses for the Future, Philadelphia, PA.

Melosh, B. (1982). *The physicians hand: Work, culture and conflict in American nursing.* Philadelphia: Temple University Press.

Mezey, M., Lynaugh, J., & Cartier, M. (Eds.) (1989). *Nursing homes and nursing care: Lessons from the teaching nursing home.* New York: Springer Publishing.

Myrdal, G. (1944). *An American dilemma.* New York: Harper and Row.

"News" (1985, September/October). *International Nursing Review, 32,* 131–137.

Nightingale, F. (1860/1969). *Notes on nursing: What it is and what it is not.* New York: Dover Publications.

Office of Technology Assessment (1986). *Nurse practitioners, physicians assistants and certified nurse-midwives: A policy analysis.* Washington, DC: U.S. Government Printing Office.

Olshansky, S. J., & Ault, A. B. (1986). The fourth stage to the epidemiologic transition: The age of delayed degenerative diseases. *The Milbank Quarterly, 64,* 355–391.

Parnell, C. (1920). The selection and organization of hospital personnel. *Transactions of the American Hospital Association, 1920.* Chicago: AHA.

"Perspectives" (1987, May 11). *Medicine and Health,* 3.

Pokorny, G. (1988). Report card on health care. *HMO First Quarter,* 3–10.

Reverby, S. (1983). Something besides waiting: The politics of private duty nursing reform in the depression. In E. C. Lagemann (Ed.), *Nursing history, new perspectives, new possibilities* (pp. 133–156). New York: Teachers College Press.

Reverby, S. (1987). *Ordered to care: The dilemma of American nursing, 1830—1945.* Cambridge, London and New York: Cambridge University Press.

Roberts, S. J. (1983, July). Oppressed group behavior: Implications for nursing. *Advances in Nursing Science, 3,* 21–22.

Rosenberg, C. (1987). *Care of strangers: The rise of America's hospital system.* New York: Basic Books.

Titus, S. C. (1952). Economic facts of life for nurses. *American Journal of Nursing, 52,* 1109–1110.

CHAPTER FOUR

Nurses' Rights

Claire M. Fagin

The word "right" is defined as a just claim to anything to which one is entitled such as power or privilege. A "right" is that which one may properly demand or claim as just, moral, or legal. A close synonym to right is prerogative.

One's rights ought to involve the creation of situations to enhance humanness. Clearly, this would include the right to exercise one's abilities, the right to express oneself freely, the right to grow *up* as well as old, the right for fair compensation for one's work, and the right to obtain satisfaction in living. Furthermore, if to humanize is to help someone become kind, merciful, considerate, civilized, and refined, some reciprocal self-enhancement is required to meet this description in relation to others. Thus, rights of humans.

NURSES' RIGHTS

What then does the fact that all human beings have the right to self expression, to full participation, and to enactment of their special

This is an updated and revised version of an article that was published in *The American Journal of Nursing,* Jan. 1975, Vol. 75, No. 1.

abilities, mean to us as nurses? What are our special rights as professionals? I would list the following rights:

1. The right to find dignity in self-expression and self-enhancement through the use of our special abilities and educational background.
2. The right to recognition for our contribution through the provision of an environment for its practice, and proper, professional economic rewards.
3. The right to a work environment which will minimize physical and emotional stress and health risks.
4. The right to control what is professional practice within the limits of the law.
5. The right to set standards for excellence in nursing.
6. The right to participate in policy making affecting nursing.
7. The right to social and political action in behalf of nursing and health care.

I believe there is a direct relationship between human rights and these nurses' rights. Human refers to whatever is descriptive of man and the word "humane" is often used to describe an expectation about the nurse. If we consider the nurse's human rights in terms of professional rights, we could list the right to be heard, the right to participate freely and effectively, the right to satisfaction, and the right to question or doubt. It is when these rights are not fulfilled, that we feel we are not being treated as human beings.

We nurses have made one clear statement of rights—the refusal to participate. To me, the *not* do, of our rights expression is significant. It's all too close to the level of learning expressed in developmental tasks where children learn who they are by saying they *don't* wish to do. This is an early step in self-development and in the differentiation aspects of who one is. I hope we can move through this step very rapidly and delineate what we have the right *to* do as well as *not* to do.

As June Rothberg (1973) has identified, our legal rights to practice and to exercise our professional rights are described in nurse practice acts and in a wealth of common law and tradition. In every state of this nation, nurses are legally responsible for their actions and inactions. A key differentiation between nurses and other legally sanctioned health professionals has to do with the public's direct access to service.

One could easily state that there is a strong relationship between such direct access and power, privilege, and rights among the health professions. Society appears to grant rights for valued service directly given rather than service delivered through an intermediary. Without this direct relationship it is difficult for the public to become aware of what a group has to offer. The public is for the most part unaware of what nursing has to offer in the improvement of health care. The public sees nursing as a sub-branch of medicine, ordered and controlled by physicians. If they have received good nursing care in a hospital, for example, they frequently believe that this is the result of physician's orders or some other control outside the realm of nursing practice and decision making.

The law in many instances tends to support this delusion, if indeed it always is a delusion. For example, in order for nurses to be paid by Medicare for their services to patients at home they must have physician's orders for any or all nursing services rendered. Although states may legalize and sanction nurses making judgments about what nursing services patients require, nurses have not been given the right to make this judgment practicable.

The New York State Nurse Practice Act, for example, states that nursing is diagnosing and treating human responses to actual or potential health problems, through such services as case finding, health teaching, health counseling, and initiation of health care. There is power and leverage within this definition. Yet few nurses have so far shown evidence of grasping this inherent power and using it effectively. Nurses, for the most part, play the role described earlier of all women—submissive, dependent, indirect, and frightened. Failure to act on behalf of our rights increases our guilt and low self-esteem and compounds our problems by discouraging the development of enabling behaviors to achieve rights. In seeking security, rather than satisfaction, we are, more often than not, unaware of our lack of achievements. Many of our constituents view their jobs as eight hours of drudgery leading, hopefully, to satisfactions in other areas of life separated from work. In this process we lose the benefits of years of education, our original motivation in becoming nurses, and the potential value of most of our awake lives.

Rather than face this misery openly and honestly we have found it much easier to focus on the responsibilities we ought to have and not have. We are more likely to blame others for the fact that we are not able to carry out the responsibilities we describe in our own nursing literature. Unfortunately, in this blaming of others we contribute to the alienation of professionals from each other and towards an ever expanding gulf of hostility and noncommunication. This is not living, no less professional practice. The highest order of *responsibility* in our priority system should be the responsibility of seeing, through unified action, that our rights are obtained. Leadership in our educational and work situations is required in order to revise the socialization process of nurses and others towards active participation and self-realization. Rigid bureaucratic settings do not encourage active participation. Nor, however, do educational settings which claim to have eliminated the trappings of bureaucracy but through covert and overt messages encourage adjustment and adaptation rather than growth and learning. It behooves us all to examine the conditions of our professional lives in order to ferret out those which inhibit self-enhancement and capitalize on aspects which will encourage our goal of advancing nurses' rights. The climate is now conducive to this goal, providing society sees itself as gaining something in return.

HOW TO KEEP RIGHTS

Nurses' rights and nurses' responsibilities come together, I believe, in the sense that frequently the carrying out of responsibilities on behalf of others will enhance our power base by increasing our support. This broadened power base helps us obtain and keep the rights nurses ought to have in health care systems. Using our rights to act politically would involve a wide range of activities calculated to affect law-making groups on behalf of direct professional interests as well as our responsibilities to the people we are serving. This kind of demand for rights, pertaining to patient care, done noisily and publicly, will help to obtain and keep the power and leverage suggested in the new definitions of nursing practice. We cannot claim what is rightfully ours unless we demonstrate some answerability for our actions. To be responsible and accountable for the delivery of nursing, we must have the authority to act and to do what is necessary to deliver this essential service. We must, through direct action, convince the public that we have a service of great value to deliver. Presently, the public's dissatisfaction with medical and hospital services harbors the threat that some long held rights of power groups may be taken away. It therefore becomes vital, in obtaining and keeping nurses' rights as professionals, to set the highest possible standards for delivering quality nursing care. Consumer validation of our view of quality nursing will clearly have an effect on our rights and legitimacy.

REFERENCE

Rothberg, J. S. (1973). *Choosing to Use Your Professional Prerogatives.* Paper presented at the Tennessee Nurses' Association Biennial Convention, held in Memphis, Tenn., Oct. 4, 1973.

CHAPTER FIVE

Executive Leadership: Improving Nursing Practice, Education, and Research

Claire M. Fagin

To find the right answers to how executive leadership can improve nursing education, practice, and research, some new questions must be raised that will better define the dilemmas in which nursing finds itself. But first, I want to examine some of assumptions underlying this chapter.

The first assumption is that nursing practice, education, and research need to be improved. **The second assumption** is that professional advances in nursing have become far too complex for one person to deal with them comprehensively. **The third assumption,** perhaps more covert than overt, is that the question of how to improve nursing education, practice, and research, which has been asked and answered hundreds of times in the past, must be looked

Note: Based on paper presented at Invitational Conference on Executive Leadership in Major Teaching Hospitals and Academic Health Centers, June 22, 1995, Cambridge, Massachusetts. It was published as an article in *Journal of Nursing Administration,* Vol. 26, No. 3, March 1996. It is reprinted here with permission.

at anew, from a different perspective, from a different context, and with a new paradigm. Thus, the answers to the question have to be different from those we have come up with before. **The fourth assumption** is that today's changes will take us into the 21st century, but I would NOT assume that we should shape our thinking on the current situation. We have seen dramatic changes in the health care field over its history and very rapid changes in the past decade. I expect that the current turmoil may be an in-between step to new solutions that will occur in a five to ten year period, as managed care is evaluated and other contemporary developments surface. **The fifth and final assumption** is that we are experiencing a crisis of national leadership in health care. Our institutions can boast of superb leaders in nursing and medicine responding to current political and managerial challenges. **But** there seems to be an absence of the visionaries, transforming nursing and medical leaders, who not only respond to their institutional challenges but also speak for their professions and for the public they serve. Such leaders help to set the national health care agenda rather than react to it.

Given these five assumptions, and particularly because of the fifth, I discuss education, practice, and research by focussing first on executive leadership in nursing. Questions are raised and recommendations are made for the here and now, and for the future.

LEADERSHIP

A useful framework for linking the worlds of the nursing educator and practitioner is Peter Senge's learning organization.[1] "A learning organization . . . is continually expanding its capacity to create its future. For such an organization, it is not enough merely to survive. 'Survival learning' . . . is important . . . But for a learning organization . . . [it] must be joined by 'generative learning,' learning that enhances our capacity to create" (p. 14). This definition is very appropriate as we examine the organizations that nurses lead. Looking at academic health centers as learning organizations suggests several questions:

1. How do we define leaders?
2. Why are we leading?
3. How do we prepare leaders?

4. Do leaders of practice disciplines such as nursing and medicine have a responsibility for building their disciplines?
5. Does nursing leadership differ from medical leadership in academic health centers?

Answers to the last question provide a distinctive picture to the nurse executive. The professions of medicine and nursing are vastly different in many aspects including their cultures, hours and patterns of work, and income expectations. Friedson defines critical aspects of a profession as its "power to control the terms, conditions, and content of its work."[2] It is this power that has been the principal differentiation between the way medicine and nursing have progressed, organized their systems, and maintained their hegemony—at least until very recently. It is probably this characteristic that influences the sharp differences in executive leadership among nursing professionals and particularly between nursing administrators in education and practice.

EDUCATIONAL ADMINISTRATORS

There are few ambiguities in the answers to my questions about leadership among nursing education administrators in major academic health centers. While particular administrative styles may differ greatly, there is clarity in the who, what, and what-for of leadership. *How do we define leaders?* When any of our institutions is searching, the desired candidate is usually described as a scholar with a track record of achievement in the discipline. That record should include some demonstrated skill in managing in a like organization, examples of influencing others in the advancement of the profession, interpersonal skills within and outside the discipline, impressive publications, and in the major academic health center world about which we are concerned here, an imposing reputation. We seek such people because we believe that the organization is in need of leadership to move the discipline forward and to represent the institution in the best way possible. From the standpoint of the faculty, they want their leader to represent them to the administration, to help them achieve their full rights and respect, to present the discipline in the most reputable way possible, and to be able to engage in the broad campus and alumni arenas in a way that brings nursing positive attention. These administrators know why they are leading. During their extensive pre-employment interviews, they give the search committee and the administration confidence that they share a creative view of leadership related to the needs of the school and discipline as well as their fit in the University.

Do we prepare academic leaders for these roles? Certainly not in any educational program I know of. One of the reasons for seeking a tested person is that learning how to use one's leadership skills comes from testing various modes of behavior in small and large venues, finding what works, seeking to develop a new and wide repertoire of responses, and evolving a persona which has enough constancy to be recognizable as one's own individual leadership style, while maintaining the flexibility to continue to develop. These administrators, in general, are awarded tenure in an academic title (not in the administrative title) on appointment, thus meeting quite clearly the professional characteristics of control and autonomy.

ADMINISTRATORS OF NURSING PRACTICE

Let me briefly address the same questions for practice leaders. While searches in academia are influenced by the higher administration or the Trustees, faculty have a major or dominant role in the choices. This differs from the practice situation where nurses in the institution play some part in the recruitment and selection; but in most institutions, a less powerful and decisive role than faculty play in universities. The expression "team players" appears in many advertisements currently, but even when this characteristic is not in print, the degree to which a candidate is a good team player is always asked when calling for references and when describing incumbents. Rarely does a Chief Executive Officer or Chief Operating Officer of an academic health center view the applicant first as a practice leader and second as a member of his or her hierarchy. Further, when the Chief Nursing Officer is a member of the School of Nursing faculty, to what degree is that role stressed in the health system search process? That answer varies with the institution, but whatever the answer, it will suggest the definition of nursing leader in the specific institution.

The cultures of academia and practice in such dimensions as control of the terms of work, autonomy, and independence, differ substantially. For the nurse executive in educational institutions there is generally parity with other professionals. For the nurse executive in service institutions the potency of professional characteristics is more cloudy and rewards in the current environment more often stress abilities to manage within a cost constrained organization over discipline building goals. There are inevitable conflicts for the nurse executive in trying to maintain and strengthen a care giving cadre of professionals in situations where the reward system is valuing that goal less than in former years.

Why are we leading? Many of our institutions are changing the role of the nursing executive. Many are adding responsibility for patient care related departments in addition to nursing; more often than not the nurse executive is the Vice President of Patient Care Services, not of nursing alone. This suggests that new answers must be given to the definition of leader and to the questions of why and who we are leading. Is the leader of nursing practice the generative and regenerative leader of nurses? Do nurse executives see themselves as increasing their scope and prestige by minimizing or, even in some cases, obliterating their nursing identification? Are nurse administrators and other nurses taking an active role in creating nursing's future? Are nurse executives reacting to the administrative and managerial hierarchies with plans for survival or with active and inspiring participation in the planning process for change? Are the responses we hear from nurses all over the country reacting to threat, rather than acting to regenerate our systems to reflect both cost and quality from the nursing frame of reference? Answers to these questions can lead to strategic actions.

Some health care institutions are substituting minimally prepared workers for nursing personnel. Others are describing new models of care utilizing cost effective health service teams but with incomplete information about the preparation of the various team members. In examining some written descriptions of these models one notes that discipline specific requirements exist only for physicians (MDs). Surely nurses exist and participate in some of the leadership roles, but the credentials do not appear. This dangerous situation appears to be part of a growing trend which has implications for the profession and for the public. For the profession, by deliberately leaving out the credential of the nursing license, nursing's power, ethic, roles, and future are made as invisible as the most stereotypic view of nursing we all decry. For the public, the potential absence of professional nurses could lead to lower quality care and in some cases to life threatening events.

These trends are of great concern. The problems nursing practice and education executives have had previously in seeking unity, will only be exacerbated by the immediate threats to the practicing nurses in these settings and the delayed, but already clear, dilemmas these changes imply for the students currently in our educational programs.

To whom must practice leaders prove themselves? As I said earlier, practice leaders do not have benefits of autonomy and control compared to education leaders. When forced into a survival mode, can practice leaders focus on building the discipline, and on the visionary, regenerative aspects of leadership? Yet this is exactly what must be done despite the difficulty of moving our mission of care forward while we respond to current crises.

Our focus must be how we move forward in a new paradigm of delivery of health services. Recognizing that our leadership role is often a position in the middle—between our staff and the administrators we also serve—our methods must include developing strategies for involving all of our nursing staff in problem solution, taking account of the present and future, and most important, recognizing that our special mission of quality nursing care must be our primary concern within the broader context. Peter Senge says that: "Most of the leaders with whom . . . [he has] worked agree that the first leadership design task concerns developing vision, values, and purpose or mission" (p. 343). Stewardship of the vision and mission is a vital function of the leader, and improvement in the three arenas of nursing education, practice, and research, requires recognition of our mutual stake in stewarding this leadership design task. There is no way that leaders in nursing education and practice can move ahead in parallel play at this time. How we work together in the strategies we design will probably tell the tale for our profession in decades ahead.

IMPROVING NURSING EDUCATION, PRACTICE, AND RESEARCH

I have advocated for some years a model of integrative nursing which includes faculty status for all appropriately credentialed practitioners in academic health centers.[3] I also believe that those faculty members whose work is predominantly in research and teaching need to be part of the health delivery arena but, perhaps, in somewhat different ways. The development of the discipline, the quality of nursing education, and the quality of nursing practice is enhanced by models which permit the pronouns "my" and "our" to be used to describe the school and health system by all nurses in the setting.

Such models require a high degree of job security so that a sense of continuity pervades the care and teaching components of the institution. For example, at the University of Pennsylvania (Penn) there is a commitment to the clinician/educator/faculty member for a period of time from the University School of Nursing. In fact, although the initial appointment may be with the University hospital, there is no requirement that this be a permanent arrangement providing that the faculty member and the School agree on a new role. Since the program started several faculty members have changed their clinical employment, most from a hospital setting to some form of community health care.

Penn's system, which grants faculty status to fully credentialed clinicians, is unusual in its flexibility and fits a variety of circumstances. It guarantees academic freedom and unites people rather than organizations.[4] At the time the system was designed downsizing of nursing personnel was not an issue. In fact, the issue at the time was how to make the hospital more attractive to nurses at all levels. Building nursing leadership through integrating practice and education was one attractive and successful strategy. Currently, downsizing nursing organizations presents questions about the potential security of hospital-based faculty positions. These questions do not lead necessarily to negative answers since the program is being maintained and enlarged.

The irony about downsizing is that its inevitability had not been planned for by the nursing community (harkening back to the leadership issues of survival versus generative leadership). A striking example of lack of foresight is that few of us took seriously the predictable outcome of the large increases in nurses' pay. Some of us warned that higher salaries would end the nursing shortage, not by recruiting new nurses but by presenting a more costly solution to hospital care than managers were willing to pay for. While it is not necessarily a bad thing to have fewer and better paid professional nurses than we were accustomed to, the nursing community did little to prepare in advance for this eventuality.

For at least four decades, goals of quality improvement have been confounded by a contradictory strategy of preparing large numbers of registered nurses at the lowest level, the two-year program, to meet the nursing needs of the public. This strategy, to produce nurses quickly to meet the needs of hospitals and nursing homes, was assumed to be sufficient to the needs of the times, attractive to a racially and ethnically diverse population, and cheap. The programs are financially supported by a wide variety of local, state, and federal funds which are not easily calculated to show cost, and, contrary to myth, the programs graduate a population less racially diverse than do baccalaureate programs. Further, nursing administrators and many educators have never urged differentiation of nurses' salaries by education so that the fast track to the RN license has led to an irrationally expensive work force based on the outworn philosophy of "a nurse is a nurse is a nurse."

While the nursing profession (among others) did not forecast the chaotic changes in health care of the mid nineties and plan its work force requirements of entry level nurses for these changes, forward looking developments were occurring at the higher end of nursing education and practice. Practice and education leaders have collaborated in building programs of innovative nursing practice in a wide variety of settings. Advanced Practice Nurses (APNs) are at the heart of these innovations. The American Association of Colleges of Nursing[5] has agreed that APNs should hold a graduate degree in nursing and be certified.

The innovations in advanced nursing practice offer us the direction in which our improvements in nursing practice and education must continue. These roles fit well with the assumptions I stated earlier and with integrated roles in schools of nursing.

Until recently, roles for APNs have been quasi independent roles, and two of them, the Nurse Practitioner(NP) and the Certified Nurse Midwife(CNM) were community roles. The newest model of the APN is a hospital based tertiary care practitioner who blends the nurse practitioner role with the clinical nurse specialist role.[6]

The Columbia-Presbyterian Medical Center in Manhattan offers two interesting examples of improved practice by implementing both the community and hospital APN roles. On selected units of the hospital, APNs do initial assessments, write admission orders, work with attending physicians to review plans of care, and with the nursing staff to interpret clinical information and explain the rationale for treatment plans. Further, APNs managing clinics in the Columbia system have admitting privileges for all of Presbyterian's hospitals. In New York, APNs have prescriptive privileges for their patients.

It's interesting that Henry Silver, Loretta Ford's co-pioneer in the nurse practitioner movement, predicted and recommended the development of a hospital-based nurse practitioner role in an article published in 1988.[7] Describing the role, he and McAtee stated, " . . . they would perform many functions and provide many services given by first-year residents in teaching hospitals" (p. 1671). They estimated that these nurses could reduce physician needs by 5–10% and reduce health care costs significantly.

NURSE SPECIALIST TRANSITIONAL CARE

It's no secret that the current payment structure for hospitals is increasingly reliant on managed care organizations. In efforts to compete for business, hospitals aim to shorten hospital stays, or eliminate hospitalization completely for many surgical procedures. Nurse specialist transitional care helps counter the fragmentation of care that many consumers experience as they navigate among different providers, treatments, and settings. Nurse-managed, hospital-based programs to provide transitional care for patients diagnosed with cancer, for perinatal care of mother and infant, for the frail elderly, for patients with AIDS, and for many other populations have been shown to be extremely effective. Many of these innovations were stimulated by the research of Dorothy Brooten[8] whose first study on early discharge of low-birthweight infants demonstrated important quality and cost results. The Brooten model has since been studied for patients with a variety of conditions who are discharged earlier from the hospital by substituting a portion of hospital care with a comprehensive program of home follow-up by APNs. Highly successful interventions have been documented for low-birth weight infants, mothers undergoing Cesarian births, high-risk mothers, women undergoing hysterectomies, and the hospitalized elderly.

Nursing has demonstrated that it can improve care for a wide variety of patients currently considered chronic or not amenable to care. For example, treatment options for patients with pain, incontinent clients, asthmatics, diabetics, and others have been initiated or assumed by nurses and are increasingly being documented. Preparation and utilization of nurses in these roles are fundamental to improvement of nursing practice and nursing education.

MANAGED CARE AND NURSE MANAGED CLINICS

We are seeing increasing interest in NPs in managed care organizations and other innovative practice settings that are community based. Day Hospitals for the elderly are nurse managed facilities, and working in tandem with hospitals and HMOs can offer appropriate care for less cost than more traditional 24-hour care or home care. We are learning that Health Maintenance Organizations and other managed care settings are relying heavily on the cost effective APN. Further, HMOs have the highest percentage of baccalaureate and higher degree nurses among employers in the U.S.[9]

Some of these nurses are in direct primary care roles. Others are in case manager roles. Under the best of circumstances, these roles can be exciting and satisfying; however, if efforts to cut costs become the paramount aim of the organization, the roles, innovative as they may be, are unsatisfying and frustrating. Further, they may conflict sharply with the values of the nursing professional. Managed care has great promise provided that it maintains a focus on the client and family and offers a strong array of services from prevention to specialty treatment.

In many parts of the United States, nurses are involved in value added roles in managed care, including those offered in the 300 (or so) nurse-managed centers throughout the nation.[10] Most of these centers offer a range of primary care, case management and wellness care. They compete with other primary care providers for clients and contracts.

School and community center clinics, expanded home health visits and work site health programs have mushroomed in recent years and utilize NPs almost exclusively. The settings may differ one from the other in the type of services and the background of the nurse provider. All stress prevention and maintenance of health. Many of them involve the community in planning and monitoring services. The notion of marketing prevention and risk reduction with vulnerable populations is implicitly or explicitly part of many nursing centers.

All of the changes we are seeing have relevance for improvement in both nursing practice and nursing education. They suggest issues and questions. Just as hospitals are changing rapidly, many of our schools are moving rapidly to prepare for the newer models of practice. Our leading centers of nursing education must focus on the kind of generative leadership necessary for their students to be able to take their places in contemporary health care with clarity about their current and changing roles and the awareness of the heavy responsibility that the nursing roles entail. To insure improvement in nursing practice and nursing education, we need to have shared answers to some vital questions. These shared answers require commitment and planning so that fragmentation and fracturing do not continue:

1. Do our academic health center schools have the faculty and clinical settings to provide a quality education for the innovative practice models developing?
2. Is there stress on nursing roles vis-à-vis prevention and maintenance of health?
3. Do our students understand the differences between case management and care management?
4. Are we preparing for the hospital environment as well as for community health settings?
5. Are we in one of our historic pendulum swings as we see the hospital market shrinking and changing in threatening ways? Are we allowing the pendulum to take precedence over long term strategies and considerations?
6. To what extent are practice and education leaders collaborating to forge a new paradigm for practice and education?
7. To what extent are practice and education leaders collaborating to sell this new paradigm to managers and administrators?
8. How are nurses uniting to examine the risks of a downsized nursing population in hospitals?

9. How are nursing practice and education leaders teaching and supporting continuity of care and accountability of nurse providers?
10. What are education and practice leaders doing in recognition of the extreme burden young nurses have in accountability and advocacy?
11. To what extent are our students and young nurses cognizant of their responsibility to protect the patient?

Whether in hospital or community care, if we lose our accountability, we lose our discipline. In recent months we have read about tragic outcomes for patients in hospitals around the country. We do not know the extent of nursing involvement in these incidents. Are we seeing a denigration of the nursing ethic of advocacy and accountability as our nursing staffs are being downsized, as our health systems' administrators downgrade the nursing role in development of generic teams, and as our chiefs of nursing services leave out the nursing word in their assumption of broader portfolios? The statement of the senior nursing officer, implicitly and explicitly, about the mission of the hospital and the principal caring profession has never been more important.

The research, education, and managerial missions are key to all of us in the health care field, but it is the nursing service mission that forms our center, gives meaning to our lives, puts us all in this frustrating and fascinating field, and must be dealt with now and not later as we move to new problems and solutions for the decades ahead. So, while I endorse completely the broader portfolio that is part of the trend for nurse executives, I urge maintaining clarity about the nursing discipline, its continued development, and its centrality to the hospital mission. The discipline and the patient will both be better served by our own clarity.

NURSING RESEARCH

The aspect of the research enterprise most germane to my central themes is: **collaboration among members of our own discipline** in the **examination and evaluation of quality of care issues**.

Let me highlight a few questions nurses and others need to be investigating under the rubric of what I will call the **bandwagon**

phenomenon. Whether we are talking about restructuring our hospitals, reengineering our universities, moving rapidly into a managed care world, virtual integration or the like, the bandwagon phenomenon seems more prevalent in the health care industry today than at any time in the past few decades. An example of questions which might be explored are:

- What evaluations are occurring with regard to rapid changes of restructuring and shifting of modalities for health care delivery?
- What are the post-hospital experiences of patients discharged earlier than formerly who do not have the expert care described by nursing researchers?
- What steps are being taken to change the culture of most managed care organizations from the healthy, young employed family to the older, and often less healthy populations they are currently seeking and for whom they are being mandated to care?
- What additional costs, if any, are being incurred as a result of a reduced Medicaid budget? E.g., are there changes in emergency room use with Medicaid and Medicare managed care organizations?

Recent reports on the last question give us cause for concern. Evaluations of the changes being made by the industry and by government are vital and are at least as much nursing's business as any other discipline's. Keeping our eye on the mission—quality patient care—what are we doing to assess change in relation to the core values of all health care providers? Some hospitals have dedicated small grant funds to help clinicians test efficacy of particular patient care interventions.[12] It would seem that the bandwagon phenomenon changes should be accompanied by funding for evaluative programs which focus not only on cost but on qualitative and quantitative results of the change. These studies will benefit from collaboration within nursing as well as between nursing and medicine.

Collaboration in the research enterprise also implies a collaborative approach to implementation of innovations into practice. What should be included among the saddest examples of dysfunctionality among nursing leaders is the poor record of implementing research-based innovations into practice. According to Bostrom and Wise,[13] a 10–15 year gap exists between discovery of potential innovations and implementation of these innovations into nursing practice. This gap is particularly troubling when it exists in one's own academic/ clinical environment. Closing this gap must move to the near top of our collective priorities.

It is crucial that we approach our future research initiatives recognizing that nursing education and nursing practice have a common agenda. Partly because of health system changes, this agenda will be shared, more often than not, with clinician/physician colleagues. Thus I would suggest that a collaborative approach with each other and with physicians is an important component of improvement of nursing research.

CONCLUSION

Improvement of nursing practice, education, and research must remain a major focus of executive nurse leaders in academic health centers. Any restructuring must include the maintenance or improvement in autonomy in the nursing roles with collaboration and interdependence in broader health care roles. Any restructuring should engage practicing nursing in job improvement and patient care improvement, not job protection. Any restructuring should address the challenge of how nursing can be positioned in academic health centers so that patient care services which are non-nursing can indeed serve patients and facilitate nurses' work in their service. Executive nurse leaders must address together the nursing workforce issues of: Reducing the production engine of the associate degree programs; recognizing the importance of nursing knowledge and skills, and how to build them and utilize them; and restructuring their nursing table of organization with an eye on both the short term and long term maintenance and building of the discipline. Improvement is not possible without extremely involved, participatory membership in problem solving of nursing colleagues representing the education and practice arenas.

So our work is cut out for us in the practice, education, and research arenas:

- Take control of our current and future destiny.
- Unite to whatever extent is possible in particular settings.

- Do not sacrifice the long term for the short term.
- Keep your eye on your mission.
- Identify where the nursing strength is in your institution and gather round that strength for forward movement. If that means giving up your own hegemony, so be it.

ENDNOTES

1. Senge, P. M. (1990). *The fifth discipline.* New York: Doubleday.
2. Friedson E. (1977). The future of professionalization. In M. Stacey (Ed.), *Health and the division of labor* (pp. 14–38). New York: Prodist.
3. Fagin, C. (1985). Institutionalizing practice: Historical and future perspectives. In *Faculty practice in action* (pp. 1–17). Washington, DC: American Academy of Nursing.
4. IBID.
5. AACN (American Association of Colleges of Nursing). (1994). *Certification and regulation of advanced practice nurses.* Washington, DC: AACN.
6. Keane, A., & Richmond, T. (1993). Tertiary nurse practitioners. *Image, 25*(4), 281–284.
7. Silver, H., & McAtee, P. (1988). Should nurses substitute for house staff? *American Journal of Nursing, 12,* 1671–1673.
8. Brooten, D., Kumar, S., Brown, L., Butts, P., Finkler, S., Bakewell-Sachs, S., Gibbons, A., & Delivoria-Papadopoulos, M. (1986). A randomized clinical trial of early hospital discharge and home followup of very low birthweight infants. *New England Journal of Medicine, 315,* 934–939.
9. Bureau of Health Professions, Division of Nursing. (1994). *The Registered Nurse Population: Findings From the National Sample Survey of Registered Nurses, March 1992.* Washington, DC: U.S. Dept. of Health and Human Services, Public Health Service, Health Resources and Services Administration.
10. Barger, S., & Rosenfeld, P. (1993). Models in community health care: Findings from a national study of community nursing centers. *Nursing and Health Care, 14*(8), 426–431.
11. Holthaus, R. (1993). Nurse-managed health care: An ongoing tradition. *Nurse Practitioner Forum, 4*(3), 128–132.
12. Franklin, P. D., Panzer, R. J., Brideau, L. P., & Griner, P. F. (1990). Innovations in clinical practice through hospital-funded grants. *Academic Medicine, 65*(6), 355–360.
13. Bostrom, J., & Wise, L. (1994). Closing the gap between research and practice. *Journal of Nursing Administration, 24*(5), 22–27.

CHAPTER SIX

Interfacing Successfully in the Interdisciplinary Group

Claire M. Fagin

Interface situations occur when the nurse executive is the only nurse on committees, boards, and other groups dealing with a wide variety of issues that may or may not be health related. Nurses are chosen by virtue of their position and reputation, and gender because a woman has been sought for such activities. Nurse executives also are often the only nurses present in interface situations with members of other disciplines in informal settings. In these as well as the more structured meetings, nurse executives need to maximize their participation so that specific and nonspecific professional goals can be advanced.

The nurse's purposes in all these contacts are multiple: 1) to advance the solution of the problems for which the group has been formed; 2) to use these important opportunities to build understanding of the profession; 3) to serve as a role model to affect stereotypical

Note: This is an updated and revised version of two articles that were published in *The Journal of Professional Nursing*, Vol. 4, No. 1 (January–February, 1988); and Vol. 4, No. 6 (November–December, 1988): pp. 395, 458. It is reprinted here with permission. The original title was "The Nurse Executive: Professional Women at the Interface, Parts 1 and 2."

thinking about nursing; 4) to advance the possibilities for nursing to maximize its effectiveness and achieve its potential; and 5) to help shape the direction of the health care system toward greater responsiveness to people's needs and abilities.

Examples of interface situations involving more than one nurse leader include a wide variety of task forces, committees, and councils dealing with both nursing and health issues. Nurses are being called on more and more to serve on important policy groups, national advisory councils, and leading positions in academic administration. Furthermore, nurses serve on corporate boards, in executive positions in nontraditional health organizations, and in state and regional health-related leadership roles. In these situations, how nurse executives deal with one another can often determine their individual or mutual success in accomplishing their goals. To accomplish their goals—whether dealing with local legislatures or the influentials who have an impact on nurses' workplaces—nurse executives must successfully communicate nursing and its issues to each specific group or individual.

One invitational conference, Nurses for the Future, was an interesting example of an interface situation. A selected group of nurse leaders engaged in dialogue with an equally selected group of health policy makers in education, economics, medicine, government, and the foundation world. Reactions of the nurses present, all articulate women and men, ran the gamut of extreme enthusiasm to depression about the conference's process and its potential outcomes. It seemed to me that the depression was caused by the response of the non-nurses to the views of some of the nurse participants about education (so what else is new?) and the inexperience of many of the nurses in dealing with this constant in the interface world.

The constancy of this type of experience is well known to those of us who have spent a great part of our professional lives trying to make a place for nursing in interdisciplinary organizations as well as advancing goals of the multiple disciplines involved. Although the depression does not go away with experience, the ability to bounce back through developing a variety of responses to expected behaviors does increase. Many such experiences allow the observer to begin to develop a gestalt of the successful behaviors of nurse executives in such forums.

Many of us are asked to recommend nurses for important groups as representatives of the profession, to provide breadth, to satisfy legislators, etc. The characteristics of the individual recommended should be considered irrespective of organizational loyalties. In the best circumstances, an individual with matching organizational loyalties, representativeness, and background can be found who also has the crucial characteristics for successful interface. The five purposes I described earlier are excellent components of an individual's success potential in an interface situation.

This area of activity—nursing's skills at handling interface situations—requires a good deal of thought from the standpoint of increasing the numbers of nurse executives who can function effectively in such roles.

There are some nonconstructive modes of behavior women and nurses often display in interface situations, including silence when non-nursing issues are being discussed; defensiveness or silence even when nursing issues are discussed; unsupportive behavior toward other women and nurses; and successful social behavior, which may mask ineffective professional participation.

I will give some examples of interface behaviors I have found useful for participation in important groups. You will undoubtedly agree with some and perhaps not with others.

Some interface groups are specific to nurse executives and include external constituencies, such as (1) local, state, or national governmental or professional agencies that serve as regulators, i.e., (a) Health Care Financing Association (HCFA), state boards, peer review organizations (PROs), and Joint Commission on Accreditation of Healthcare Organizations (JCAHO) and (b) professional organizations such as Council of Teaching Hospitals (COTH), National League for Nursing (NLN), and other accrediting groups; and (2) committees, consumer or otherwise, boards or voluntary agencies or corporations, government task forces, etc. Other important interface groups are internal constituencies such as trustees, medical boards, executive committees, personnel committees, and other schools in an institution.

I believe the necessary skills for successful participation in interface relationships include (1) the art of initiating, developing, and maintaining contacts; (2) an appropriate mix of personal, social, and professional interests; and (3) the ability to project a successful, knowledgeable, and energetic image.

Interpersonal competence is, by definition, the basis for all of these skills. It is the skill or set of abilities that allows an individual to shape the responses he or she elicits from others. Correctly predicting the impact of one's own actions on another person's definition of the situation, having a varied and large repertoire of possible lines of action, and using the necessary interpersonal resources to employ appropriate tactics are components of interpersonal competence.[1] The art of interpersonal competence is a vital characteristic of leadership.

Clearly, interpersonal competence is developmental in nature. Thus, gaining experience, maturity, adaptability, openness, and self-confidence will contribute to increased interpersonal competence. A person with these skills would be articulate and comfortable with a range of issues; able to deal with persons of varied status; at ease in his or her own situation, in broad professional situations at home, and internationally; and both politic and political.

My specific guidelines for interface situations follow:

(1) Be prepared to speak knowledgeably on at least one, and preferably more, non-nursing issues on every agenda at every meeting. Never allow yourself to be silent at a meeting. Read some high-quality professional nursing and non-nursing journals; the *New England Journal of Medicine*, at least one business magazine or the *Wall Street Journal*; and a newspaper the caliber of the *New York Times*.

(2) Support colleagues in your own and other disciplines about their issues. You will want such support someday and you won't get it if you don't give it.

(3) Be visible or ensure that other nurses are in relation to political candidates or volatile issues of the day (e.g., mayoral campaigns, nuclear and peace issues, acquired immune deficiency syndrome [AIDS]).

(4) Put your money where your mouth is. What counts in your community? In your institution? Who are the power brokers? Are you there working alongside them? Determined visibility, when politic, is always correct.

(5) *Never* use the sexual approach to make or win points (e.g., clothing, hair, mannerisms).

(6) Finally, always keep your eye on the *principle*, while being able to compromise on the level of strategy.

ENDNOTE

1. Foote, N., & Cottrell, L. (1955). *Identity and interpersonal competence.* Chicago: University of Chicago, pp. 41–42.

CHAPTER SEVEN

Nursing and Consumerism

Claire M. Fagin and Leah F. Binder

Today there is widespread consensus among health providers and consumer interests that health promotion and disease prevention are vital elements in a high-quality, cost-effective health care delivery system. Numerous campaigns dealing with one or another health problem are ongoing or episodic. But consensus splits on the question of how to most effectively convince consumers to respond to these campaigns by altering behaviors.

The delivery system as it is currently structured contains few incentives for providers to contribute to preventive and/or promotional efforts. On the contrary, the health care system frequently offers incentives for implementation of high-technology, high-skill operations, procedures, and interventions without addressing the preventive mechanisms that would eliminate some of the demand for such services.[12] As a result, millions of Americans have little contact with the health care system until they land in the emergency room, and millions more partake in dangerous behaviors—such as failing to obtain appropriate vaccinations or continuing sexual encounters

Note: This was originally published as a chapter in Joanne McCloskey and Helen Grace, *Current Issues in Nursing*, Mosby, St. Louis, 1988, 450–459. It is reprinted here with permission.

when suffering from a sexually transmitted disease—that could be discouraged with appropriate noncoercive professional help.[31] This chapter will examine effective efforts to provide for the public health—both within the context of the health care delivery system and outside—and recommend strategies for change that involve integrating consumers more fully into the decision-making fabric of the health care system.

It is important to recognize that despite its flaws, health care in the United States is not without successes in the arena of preventive and promotional health. Efforts to discourage smoking have resulted in the decline in smoking among Americans, and attempts to encourage behaviors that defend against heart disease, such as healthier diets and exercise, have similarly shown promise. Nonetheless, on key international indicators of health quality, notably longevity and infant mortality, the United States competes poorly with other industrialized nations despite health expenditures second to none.[15] There is much more work ahead, and for a variety of reasons, nurses are in a unique position to forge the way forward.

BACKGROUND

In 1984 I (Fagin) was fortunate enough to have been granted one of the first two Distinguished Scholar Awards from the American Nurses' Foundation for a project to investigate the links between nursing and consumerism. I set out to develop a model of effective collaboration between organized consumers and nursing. What emerged from this project were two welcome surprises. First, although it seemed at the start that consumers and nurses might have distinct goals in health care that might not be congruent—nurses seeking to advance the profession, consumers aiming for self-help within or without the health system—it soon became clear that the two groups shared very powerful common interests with explosive potential. Indeed, the origins of the nursing profession in the United States were influenced to a large extent by consumer involvement. The influence of volunteers in hospital schools of nursing was extremely important, and the quality of schools was often a direct result of the priorities these women placed on service, training, and student life.[23]

An intraorganizational collaboration that could be said to be a direct historical antecedent of the current project was the National Organization for Public Health Nursing (NOPHN).

> Consumer involvement was an integral part of the philosophy on which NOPHN was founded. Lay membership—at first non-voting, but very soon fully participatory—was considered a radical idea, but the insistence of the NOPHN on inclusion of lay members was based on the belief that nursing is a problem of the community as well as of the profession. [Though] early activities of lay members were heavily slanted toward fund-raising, their responsibilities were constantly broadened as time went on and soon included policy-setting and directional areas.[5]

In 1952 seven organizations decided that they could best be served by a single organization "in which nurses and others interested in health services could work together." The National League for Nursing was composed of nurses, allied professionals, and interested citizens as individual members, and of nursing schools and public health nursing agencies as agency members. Of the nurse members, only those who had belonged to NOPHN had previous collaborative experience as equals with nonnurses.[25] NOPHN's 40-year history provided convincing evidence of the strength of collaboration between nurses and nonnurses both in the development of nursing as a community service and in improving the welfare of society.

The volunteer tradition, and the organizational experience of the NOPHN laid the groundwork for collaborative activities that were to come in the fields of mental health, maternal health and midwifery, child health, hospice care, and other significant movements in service and education—which became the second surprise finding in my study. The extent to which nurses and consumers were collaborating in a variety of effective initiatives was remarkable, and it provided a framework of past success that I believe offers insight as we move forward with new collaborative efforts.

Today, perhaps no group of nurses has stronger organized ties with consumers than nurse-midwives. There is no question that one of the reasons for the success of midwives in achieving reimbursement earlier than other nurses is the consumer desire for midwives' care. Consumers faced with the threat of having midwife services curtailed collaborate with each other and with midwives to pressure for their choice of services. Because midwife services are reimbursed, more people are able to experience this care and hence strengthen their preference for these kinds of services.

One of the initiatives I examined that exemplified this support for midwifery was Consumers for Choices in Childbirth, a citizens' action group that arose from the need to support midwives' practice at Yale in the late fall of 1976. The Yale nurse-midwifery practice began in 1975 with an agreement with Yale's department of obstetrics and gynecology. Not anticipating that the practice would be extremely successful, there was considerable surprise about the number of clients interested in the practice and subsequently a lack of interest on the part of physicians in serving as consultants or backups to the practice. When complaints came from clients about the discontinuity of medical consultation, the department of obstetrics and gynecology decided to close the practice. Much to the surprise of physicians, the decision to close the practice created havoc in the community. There was an outpouring of consumer sentiment regarding midwives and expressions of great enthusiasm about their care. The clients involved in the consumer coalition made it clear that their concerns had to do with consistent obstetrical consultation that was supportive of midwifery care.

Citizen outrage at physicians' derogatory remarks about clients of midwifery services and about the midwives was channeled into constructive, assertive behaviors to enable others to receive the high-quality care they had received from the midwives in the past. The committee sent letters, circulated petitions, and elicited support from others by publishing a newsletter to report their activities. They discussed issues of importance to pregnant women and parents, and sent representatives to the health systems agency. The midwifery practice was reinstated with adequate physician backup.[4]

In other areas of nursing care, people have not been as likely to establish a preference for health care provided by nurses because information and reimbursement are not as readily available. This is changing, however, for two reasons. First, the growth of managed care and preferred provider arrangements has frequently entailed increased employment of nurse practitioners and clinical nurse specialists to provide ongoing, primary health care and other services.[22] Second, state and federal reimbursement laws are changing, and nurses may now practice autonomously in many rural areas and selected additional sites. In response to the expansion of consumer access to direct nursing services, the linkages between consumers and nurses on the political and individual levels have become more sophisticated and more identifiable in the seven years since I first examined collaborative opportunities between nurses and consumers.

The best example of the growth in consumer-nurse relations is embodied by one nurse, Terry Chalich, RN. In the early 1980s, on her own time and funds, Chalich developed a program to help unemployed workers find health care.[24] Her belief that nurses have a great responsibility in dealing with the present health care crisis was translated into action: Not only did she volunteer but she stimulated volunteerism within her community and among her colleague providers. She set up offices where providers offer free or low-cost care, established a resource list of other health care services for the unemployed, disseminated literature outlining help available to the unemployed, and even negotiated with hospital billing offices to reduce fees. Chalich's network proved very successful in meeting critical needs in her community, and it earned her a strong reputation in the community. In 1990 Chalich was an unsuccessful candidate for Congress, but she was successful in raising issues in nursing and health care reform. In a 1992 article describing her campaign, Chalich[2] identified other nurse activists involved in community change, among them Sharon Malhotra, who has taken national leadership in exposing risks associated with lawn care pesticides.

THE CHALLENGE BEFORE US

My study and subsequent developments indicate that bringing nurses together with consumers on the political and community level works best when consumers are already organized and informed, and when nurses are both active participants and knowledgeable resources moving forward with consumers in the same direction. This train is on the tracks and rolling.

Currently, one of the problems of involving consumers actively in decision making is that public health campaigns—efforts to encourage healthy lifestyles—are often considered in isolation from the experience of consumers within the entire health care delivery system. Part of the reason for separating the two issues has been that different people dominate in the two aspects of health efforts: Coalitions of professionals and lay people from a variety of backgrounds—from social workers to public health specialists to community leaders—tend to advance public health campaigns, while the delivery setting is more hierarchical and dependent on perceived professional status. Nurses tend to be present as leaders and/or experts in both contexts.

In fact, from the nursing perspective, public health campaigns and the delivery setting are not separate spheres of action but interrelated agendas, and the problems of the delivery setting plague public health movements. At the heart of the problem is the medical model and consequent public mythology about the role of the delivery system. According to the myth, which has been portrayed in numerous media outlets, the health care system consists of an assembly of physicians who take charge of people's lives when an unfortunate incident occasions the need for a cure. Occasionally the cure is not forthcoming, but often enough physicians are able to stem the tide of tragic consequence. Either way, the physician, and the health care system he or she represents, is an episodic occurrence that retreats into oblivion once the cure issue is settled.[30] What people discover when they encounter the real health care system is that the majority of providers are not physicians, the majority of health care needs are not amenable to cure, and the majority of consumers should be availing themselves of some form of regular, as opposed to episodic, contact with providers.

The contrast between the myth and the reality has in the past proved difficult for Americans to accept, or even acknowledge. Perri Klass[9] received angry letters and even a death threat when she noted in her memoirs of medical residency that most people admitted to a hospital cannot be cured. The concept that, for all its impressive accomplishments, medical science is severely limited in scope troubled many of her readers. The image of the kindly physician dispensing problem-solving drugs and cures is so powerful that it is the image most parents encourage their children to view as reality and take for granted as the building block relationship at the foundation of the health care system.

It is not quite like believing in Santa Claus to believe in physicians like Marcus Welby and the medical model he exemplifies, because some physicians and medical interventions clearly save lives and make people feel better. Even health problems that do respond to medical interventions, however, are not treated with provider intervention alone. On the contrary, no broken leg will become whole, no disease will enter remission, no wound will heal without the preeminent authority and power of the human body. Diseases like acquired immunodeficiency syndrome (AIDS), which attack the body's immune system, demonstrate in tragic ways the limits of medical science—not only medicine's inability to cure the particular virus, but also medicine's inability to fend off disease in the absence of bodily mechanisms that enable interventions to work.

But the fact that providers merely assist the body in healing itself has been obscured by the romanticized concept that providers are in charge of the curative function. The power dynamic implicit in the idealized doctor-patient relationship is a dominant-subordinate one, and as a result the idealized role of health care consumers negotiating the health care system has been a subordinate, passive role. For the consumer, interaction with the health care system becomes an exercise in vulnerability and even humility, rather than a consultation with professionals on achieving one's optimal health. The results are often unhealthy: Some consumers avoid health services until the last possible moment; others do the opposite, compulsively clinging to health providers expecting cures for myriad often-undefinable ailments.

Thus the challenge for improving the public health goes beyond imparting information about healthy lifestyles, preventive care, or even quality of care. At its roots, the challenge of public health calls for consumer participation as full partners in the health care system, actively responsible for their own ongoing health maintenance and vigilant in demanding quality and cost effectiveness. This is the nursing model of care.

PROMOTING CHANGE

Recently, significant changes have occurred that indicate progress will be rapid in the coming decade toward a more powerful role for consumers. Our health care system is in the midst of revolutionary change. Contributing to this are an increasingly older population;

necessary changes in primary focus away from cure to care because of lowered mortality rates and higher morbidity and chronicity; changing values regarding who gets how much care, permitting major reallocations of economic risk; alternative health care systems and providers; and extraordinary growth in for-profit health care in segments of the enterprise. The consumer as represented by the large employer or corporation can and has exercised considerable clout in these enormous changes.

But the process has only begun. Numerous factors, such as the unusually high rate of unnecessary surgeries and procedures,[32] suggest that consumer vigilance and other regulatory checks and balances are not what they should be. Most important for the public health will be a philosophical change on the part of the consumer with regard to the locus of control in health matters: Away from the physician to the consumer, with the simultaneous development of personal accountability for one's health and medical choices. This will require change in fundamental aspects of human behavior. Such a challenge cannot be underestimated. Changing behaviors and mind-sets, even when they are clearly in the self-interest of targeted populations, is an agenda that has perplexed governments and philosophers since Stone Age policymakers tried to induce people to use the wheel.

However, a positive shift in public attitudes is occurring that may mean a change in the way people perceive health care in their lives. Numerous public opinion polls demonstrate increased distrust of the health care system and vigilance on the part of consumers in evaluating the health care they are receiving,[18] which may mean fewer passive, "doctor knows best" patients in the future. Consumers are also acting on the political level to enforce change in the delivery system. Groups such as the American Association of Retired Persons (AARP) and the National Consumers' League emerged from relative obscurity to become by the mid-1980s major forces in national health policy making.[28] Some congressional campaigns have in recent times turned on the candidate's position on health reform.[7]

EMPOWERING COMMUNITIES

As we examine strategies for achieving transition in the public posture with regard to health care, it is instructive to bear in mind the social and political context in which significant change must occur. Policymakers are approaching questions of social welfare differently than in the past, which will likely have an impact on the outcome and velocity of health care reform. They are important strategies for nurses to consider.

The 1992 riot in Los Angeles, sparked by what was widely perceived as a racist verdict in a police excessive-force case, killed more than 50 people, injured hundreds more, and resulted in millions of dollars worth of damage to inner-city communities. In the wake of the riot, partisan accusatory fingers began assigning blame. From Republicans came an attack on the Great Society programs begun in the Johnson administration, which pundits on the right accused of creating and sustaining a "culture of dependency" among inner-city residents;[10] from Democrats arose denouncement of the Reagan and Bush administrations' cuts to federal entitlement and urban development programs that, claimed the left, exacerbated poverty and hopelessness in the community.[21]

In some sense, both sides were correct: lack of federal attention in the 1980s to urban poverty contributed to community decay, and at the same time the approach of the Great Society programs has tended to disempower those it was intending to serve. But partly in the process of rebuilding Los Angeles, new ideas arose about the role of the public and private sectors in stimulating growth, opportunity, and hopefulness in poor areas. In a best-selling book published around the time of the Los Angeles riot, David Osborne and Ted Gaebler exemplified the new thinking by identifying models of what they called "entrepreneurial governments," which

> promote competition between service providers. They empower citizens by pushing control out of the bureaucracy, into the community. They measure the performance of their agencies, focusing not on inputs but on outcomes. They are driven by their goals—their missions—not by their rules and regulations. They redefine their clients as customers and offer them choices. . . . They prevent problems before they emerge, rather than simply offering services afterward. . . . And they focus not simply on providing public services, but on catalyzing all sectors—public, private, and voluntary—into action to solve their community's problems.[14]

According to this model, governments steer rather than row,[19] lending direction and support to local communities, citizens, businesses, and nonprofit organizations, which are then responsible for providing the substantive essence of community needs. Instead of direct services, governments will move toward more participatory government models.

The Osborne and Gaebler model was applied, though not deliberately, by columnist and politician Alan Keyes, who suggested that inner-city development must begin by empowering neighborhoods and communities to create their own governing bodies that would administer social welfare programs, operate a sheriff's department, and authorize a community justice of the peace. The most important weakness of many poor communities, said Keyes, "may be the fact the community itself has no authority over the many government programs that affect its individual inhabitants. Because of this deficiency there is no connection between the help the individual receives and the decent mores the community needs to encourage."[8] When responsible citizens in a community have some authority to regulate conditions and rules in the neighborhood, adds Keyes, youngsters are provided with constructive, instead of destructive, role models. Communities set their own standards and enforce them through peer pressure as well as laws.[8]

PUBLIC HEALTH IN THE COMMUNITY

The approach of the reinvented government model mirrors in many respects the recommendations of Nursing's Agenda for Health Care Reform. Nurses, too, recommend shifting activity away from large acute care settings and toward smaller community settings for the delivery of health services, and encouraging a free-market competitive environment by revealing to consumers information and data about quality of care not previously available.[17] In the end, the philosophical approach of nursing's agenda and the reinvented government model are identical: Empower citizens by creating avenues of participation, and promote higher accountability between providers and recipients of services.

The dual issues of citizen empowerment and community-level approaches to policy making offer important possibilities for meeting public health needs and ought to guide us as we formulate a model for bringing consumers into the fold. The community-based perspective appears to be a major determinant in the success of public health efforts. For example, a wide-ranging analysis of three studies that investigated community-based cardiovascular disease prevention programs found that when practitioners gained collaboration from residents and community leaders, the campaigns could be effective.[14] Numerous other examinations of the trend toward health promotion in the community have revealed similar positive results. An analysis of the trend by communications specialist John L. McKnight concludes by recommending continued efforts on the community level, pointing out that "to enhance community health, we need a new breed of modest health professional. They are people with a deep respect for the integrity and wisdom of citizens and their associations."[13]

Luckily, the members of this "new breed" of unassuming, respectful health professionals qualified to provide care at the community level are graduating from nursing school—and practicing for years in a variety of settings in communities across America. Indeed, nurses are active participants in many of the most successful community health campaigns.

The definition of community need not be limited to precise neighborhood parameters. In a study conducted by Motivational Educational Entertainment, investigators found that teenagers in inner-city neighborhoods in Philadelphia; Camden, New Jersey; New York; Washington, D.C.; and Oakland, California, had been raised in a milieu so removed from American mainstream culture that no medium except rap music was credible enough to convey effective messages on improving or escaping life in the ghetto.[34] Researchers explained that the youth "have leaders, a social structure" and derided national public service campaigns aimed at curbing drug use or advocating safer sex practices as "mainstream assumptions that these are rudderless, leaderless young people yearning for a catch phrase upon which to focus their lives."[34] Researchers believed that rap music represented a way to reach inner-city teens on their own terms, within the reputation of the community they identified with—a larger national community of black, alienated teens. The public health message could only reach them through the avenues defined as most reputable within that community.

Another community without walls is the gay community, which has responded in exemplary ways to the scourge of the AIDS epidemic. According to the Centers for Disease Control, community demonstration projects revealing the most positive changes in sex practices were in "cities with strong gay communities and positive images of gay men."[20] Unfortunately, this is one bright spot within a discouraging context. Studies on the national level indicate a large proportion of individuals with AIDS remain sexually active,[26] and studies by the National Institutes of Health and the Centers for Disease Control suggest that knowledge of human immunodeficiency virus (HIV) status does not in itself produce appropriate behavioral change.[20] Thus the community structure and its propensity to accept a new message are vital links in efforts to promote healthful behaviors.

TARGETED CAMPAIGNS FOR HEALTH PROMOTION

Why does the community presence appear to correlate with the impact of public health ventures? In part the reason is rooted in classical understanding of effectiveness in public health campaigns, which was described most efficaciously by investigators in a Stanford study on the role of communications in health. Researchers concluded that possession of favorable attitudes about the message of a public health campaign does not in itself ensure the adoption of the practice recommended: people need in addition the skills and resources to undertake a behavioral modification. "It is essential in planning any health intervention to consider kinds of changes expected," the researchers warned. "Be skeptical of any health program that assumes that informing people will be enough to win their cooperation."[27] The study cited the example of smoking cessation campaigns: programs that point out the gravity of the health risk have limited success; programs that advise and assist smokers on the process of living without cigarettes may see better results.[27]

The problem of providing an effective solution-based approach to health promotion may explain the difficulty of national or broad-based mass media campaigns. Campaigns that simply offer information about a health problem are likely to have minimal impact, but the state of the art in public health is advanced enough that these are now relatively rare. Most campaigns are instead designed to advise people on taking steps to solve the identified problem. But broad-based campaign recommendations have to straddle a fine line between on the one hand offering broad advice applicable to a wide variety of targeted audiences and on the other hand offering some form of step-by-step approach that appears to be most effective in altering behaviors. The specified, step-by-step approach runs the risk of being too narrow in focus to apply to a diverse audience; the broad approach might not be helpful to anyone.

This problem of recommending practicable behaviors for a diverse audience has plagued many mass media campaigns. A study of mass media antismoking campaigns in Australia aimed at informing smokers of risks and suggesting they avoid smoking concluded that while the campaigns managed to educate people of the health risks, they did not appear successful in convincing people to quit.[11] Another study with similarly discouraging results was conducted by psychologists in South Carolina who examined the effects of an alcohol education presentation aimed at adolescents. Though the tenth and eleventh grade students in the study exhibited enhanced knowledge of the topic, there was no observable change in attitudes or alcohol involvement.[13]

Mass media campaigns that include detailed recommendations for consumer response have shown success. A campaign in Connecticut offered low-cost screening mammograms to women over the age of 34 who had not been previously examined, and it resulted in 2500 inquiries over a 7-day period.[6] In Australia investigators examined the outcome of a television show that gave instructions on recognizing signs of melanoma and recommended visiting a physician if signs were present. An increase of 167% was observed in the number of melanomas diagnosed in the 3 months after the show was aired, including a significant shift in the proportion of tumors removed in the thin, easily treated stage.[29]

Another mass media campaign that appears to have demonstrated remarkable success is the "designate a driver" campaign of the Harvard School of Public Health.[1] Utilizing a variety of mass media outlets, including public service announcements and entertainment media, the campaign has been effective because it offers a solution to the problem of drunk driving that is specific, memorable, and applicable to most populations. A broader approach to the problem of drunk driving might be "don't drink and drive," or the even broader "don't drink," which are clearly difficult for consumers to undertake when alcohol consumption is a problem. The Harvard campaign thus narrowed its focus to suggest a simple, relatively easy way to address the problem that would likely be workable for virtually every audience reached by the mass media. The slogan also made its way into the cultural language and thus achieved some community reinforcement.[1]

It seems obvious there is a need for practical public health campaigns targeted with recommendations for action that specific populations will be able to access. The community-based model would likely be able to target particular identified populations more efficiently and directly than the mass media strategy, which is an important component of effective public health efforts. While health problems in and of themselves do not usually vary from a purely scientific point of view, the behavioral changes and personal initiatives required of populations facing the challenges are often vastly different. For instance, family planning in a poor inner-city neighborhood requires different kinds of services and counseling than in a suburban middle-class community.

Thus many public health initiatives may prove most effective when targeted to meet the specific needs and skill levels of particular populations and aimed at introducing practical solutions to health problems. People may also be less resistant or distrustful of the message when conveyed within the community, using reputable community outlets (such as rap music to reach inner-city teens). Furthermore, participation within the community in reinforcing behavioral change can, as previously discussed, be a powerful catalyst for behavioral change. Researchers at the University of New Mexico School of Medicine conducted an analysis of the literature on community-based public health and examined case studies to propose a model of "empowerment education," which suggests participation of people in group action and dialogue efforts directed at community targets and shows considerable promise.[33]

INFORMATION AND EMPOWERMENT

Information about health promotion is not the only kind of information consumers need to become powerful participants in their own health maintenance. Consumers also need knowledge of the health system, its constraints, its options, varieties of insurance benefits available, and cost-effective providers, as well as information about the most common health problems affecting them in their age group and appropriate self-care. Consumers should be informed about known evidence of outcome of procedures and operations they consider, and have access to information they need to select providers and settings on the basis of qualitative criteria. We cannot make intelligent choices in a competitive health care system without such information being widely available through an array of media and spokespersons. Ultimately, without a range of information, consumers cannot effectively pressure for change, because it is difficult to know which changes are beneficial to them and which are not.

But just like information provided for health promotion purposes, the availability of information about the range of options in the delivery setting depends on the willingness of consumers to do something with the new knowledge. Will consumers exercise the power of the purse to create the changes necessary in the delivery system? Will they use information about quality to choose appropriate providers and settings? Will they demand changes in the delivery setting and outside it that will refocus health care toward the real needs of consumers? Will they move from the prescribed mythological role of passive recipient of cure to the powerful role of participant and guardian of their own health?

NURSES: STEERING TOWARD CONSUMER EMPOWERMENT

The role suggested for "reinvented government" of (1) steering but not rowing, (2) emphasizing prevention of crisis, and (3) being mission-driven in our approach to public business applies to nurses interested in reinventing health care. As consumers achieve new confidence and competence in negotiating health care, evaluating options, and maintaining their own health, nurses have an unusual opportunity to move consumers toward empowerment—not by achieving it for them, but by steering consumers forward. We can do this in a variety of ways. First, in advancing Nursing's Agenda for Health Care Reform, we advocated positioning nurses as "gatekeepers" within the delivery setting, monitoring prescribed care regimens across providers and settings, and aiding consumers in choosing among recommended procedures, prescriptions, and care.[17] In this position, nurses can function as patient advocates, translating complex information into concrete options and formulas for consumer decision making. The consumer makes the decision, but nurses are in the position of (1) spearheading consumer usage of valuable information, which if implemented on a widespread basis would likely lead to innovations in the delivery setting aimed at enhancing efficiency, quality, and cost effectiveness and (2) discouraging on a mass scale the habits of patient subordination that are ingrained in consumers and perpetuated in part by the current health system structure.

Nurses are also challenged on the community level to continue the innovations in health promotion and create new models for health service delivery that will reach the public more effectively. This is especially true in poor communities, where access to health services is often extremely limited, but it is equally valuable for middle-class communities, where cost-effective health services and enhanced consumer vigilance are also needed.

Consumer-nurse alliances at the community level are feasible, desirable, and, as we have seen from the efficacy of community-level action in general, strategically effective. When starting such a coalition, it is best to begin with one or two specific goals, instead of a broad agenda. Goals might include any of the following:

- *Releasing information about quality of care.* A community group could dedicate itself to publicly revealing information about the quality of care delivered by local hospitals, nursing homes, community health care agencies, and private practice providers. Some information, such as hospital mortality data, is readily available.* Most critical information is not released to the public, however, and a community-based coalition to press for announcement of key quality indicators might succeed not only in unveiling hidden information of import, but also in imple-

---

*For information on hospital mortality rates contact: Health Care Financing Administration, Office of Public Affairs, www.HCFA.gov.

menting a campaign to politically involve consumers in the policies and procedures of health care delivery.

- *Promoting the public health—healthy lifestyles.* A number of initiatives, such as smoking cessation, fitness, and disease prevention, are excellent targets of community campaigns. The key, as discussed earlier, is to suggest alternative behaviors to targeted populations and then help them access these alternatives to the extent possible.

- *Setting up community nursing centers.* There are community nursing centers in hundreds of communities from California to New York.[16] These centers use innovative approaches to encouraging citizen participation in the process of delivering health care within the community with promising results.[16] Some are private practice arrangements with nurses providing direct care; others are affiliated with nursing schools, hospitals, or other agencies to provide care in the community. Some target particular populations, such as the elderly or adolescents, while others provide a variety of services to a broad population. There are a variety of funding options available to help nurses start community nursing centers, including foundation support, federal and state grants, and university subsidies. Nurses seeking to start a center should start at the level of the community they intend to serve, connecting with citizen groups that might be interested in helping get a center off the ground. The community nursing center is the essence of Nursing's Agenda for Health Care Reform and is almost exclusively advanced at the community level.

- *Advancing nursing's agenda for health care reform.* Nursing's agenda does not exist in a vacuum. It is wholly dependent upon citizen support and initiative on its behalf—and the community will again be critical in that effort. A coalition of groups and/or individuals interested in promoting the agenda could hold functions and speaking engagements to discuss the agenda's approach to various issues of concern to the community's health needs. A community with a large elderly population might be interested in how increased access to home care services might affect citizens in the community; a younger population might explore options in the agenda for prenatal care provided by nurses.

All community consumer-nurse collaborative efforts should aim to generate not only increased general knowledge about possibilities in health care, but actual changes in the way health care is experienced in communities. Build a center. Start a home care agency. Create a new insurance plan for local employers to buy into. While in many cases state and federal laws will restrict creation of new models, it is important that communities try to bang down the legal doors slammed shut on communities suffering from health hazards that are preventable, treatable, and/or affordably dealt with.

Ultimately, by maintaining a presence in schools, community centers, and communities throughout the nation, and upholding the nursing model of care that specifies patient empowerment and respect for individuality, nurses can break the model of dominant-subordinate provider-patient relations that has discouraged so many Americans from utilizing the system appropriately.

The time is ripe for transformation in the health care system that will bring consumers into the fold as equals in the delivery of health care and leaders in the promotion of their own care. It will be up to nurses and others to couple health promotion efforts and traditional public health messages with a campaign to empower consumers within the delivery system and expose the mythology of enforced passivity that many Americans believe is endemic to receiving health services. So far only nurses have stepped forward to promote such changes in the delivery of health care.

Nurses have traditionally viewed clients as equals—partners in the delivery of health care, not subordinates to be given orders. We must continue to take that philosophy into American communities and into Congress. Given the emerging role of consumers individually, within communities, and nationally, the potential for change is enormous, and nurses will be instrumental in its effectiveness.

ENDNOTES

1. Carter, B. (1989, September 11). Television: A message on drinking is seen and heard. *New York Times.*
2. Chalich, T., & Smith, L. (1992). Nursing at the grassroots. *Nursing and Health Care, 13,* 242–244.

3. Collins, D., & Cellucci, T. (1991, August). Effects of a school-based alcohol education program with a media prevention component. *Psychology Reports, 69,* 191–197.
4. Fagin, C. (1984). *A model for the effective collaboration between organized consumers and nursing—Report of an American Nurses' Foundation sponsored project.* Unpublished report.
5. Fitzpatrick, L. (1975). *The National Organization for Public Health Nursing (NOPHN) 1912–1952: Development of a practice field* (pp. 163–164). New York: National League for Nursing.
6. Gregario, D. I., Ikegeles, S., Parker, C., & Benn, S. (1990, July). Encouraging screening mammograms: Results of the 1988 Connecticut breast cancer detection awareness campaign. *Connecticut Medicine, 54,* 370–373.
7. Its eye on election, White House to propose health care changes. (1991, November 12). *New York Times.*
8. Keyes, A. (1992, June 8). Restoring community. *National Review, 44*(11), 38–41.
9. Klass, P. (1987). *A not entirely benign procedure: Four years as a medical student.* New York: Putnam.
10. Kramer, M. (1992, May 18). Two ways to play the politics of race. *Time, 139,* 35–36.
11. Macaskill, P., Pierce, J. P., Simpson, J. M., & Lyle, D. M. (1992, January). Mass media-led anti-smoking campaign can remove the education gap in quitting behavior. *American Journal of Public Health, 82,* 96–98.
12. Maraldo, P. (1989, Fourth Quarter). The nursing solution. *Health Management Quarterly,* pp. 18–19.
13. McKnight, J. L. (1992, February 6). Remarks made at the Medicine for the 21st Century Forum conference, sponsored by the American Medical Association and the Corporation for Public Broadcasting, Rancho Mirage, Calif.
14. Murray, D. (1992, February 6). *Lessons learned from the NLHBI sponsored community based cardiovascular disease prevention studies.* Paper presented at the Medicine for the 21st Century Forum conference, Rancho Mirage, Calif.
15. National Center for Health Statistics. (1988). *Vital statistics 1988.* Rockville, MD: U.S. Department of Health and Human Services, Public Health Services.
16. National League for Nursing. (1992, May 13). *Community nursing centers: A promising new trend in American health.* Paper presented at the National League for Nursing conference, Washington, D.C.
17. National League for Nursing & American Nurses Association. (1991). *Nursing's agenda for health care reform.* New York: Author.

18. *New York Times/CBS News health care poll.* (1991, August 18–22). Storrs, Conn: Roper Center.

19. Osborne, D., & Gaebler, T. (1992). *Reinventing government: How the entrepreneurial spirit is transforming the public sector.* New York: Addison-Wesley.

20. Patton, C. (1990). *Inventing AIDS* (p. 29). New York: Routledge.

21. Race against time. (1992, May 25). *New Republic, 206,* 7–9.

22. Schull, D., Tosch, P., & Wood, M. (1992). Clinical nurse specialists as collaborative care managers. *Nursing Management, 23,* 30–34.

23. Sheahan, D. (1981, May 22–23). *Influence of occupational sponsorship on the professional development of nursing.* Paper presented at the conference on the history of nursing to Rockefeller Research Center, Pocanizo-Hills, N.Y.

24. Sleby, T. L. (1984). RN helps unemployed find health services that are affordable. *American Nurse, 16,* 1–24.

25. Sleeper, R. (1972). *Changing years of National League for Nursing, 1952–1972.* New York: National League for Nursing.

26. Smith, H. L., Peragallo, N., Ferrer, X., Lake, E. T., & Aiken, L. H. (1987). *AIDS prevention research: Population-based and epidemiological perspectives, as applied to the AIDS epidemic in Chile.* Interim report.

27. Solomon, P., McAnany, E., Goldschmidt, D., Parker, E., & Foote, D. (1979, January). *The role of communication in health. Stanford University Institute for Communications Research.* Washington, DC: U.S. Agency for International Development.

28. Starr, P. (1982). *Social transformation of American medicine.* New York: Basic Books.

29. Theobald, T., Marks, R., Hill, D., & Dorevitch, A. (1991, October). Goodbye sunshine: Effects of a television program about melanoma on beliefs, behavior, and melanoma thickness. *Journal of the American Academy of Dermatology, 25,* 717–723.

30. Turow, J. (1989). *Playing doctor: Television, storytelling, and medical power.* New York: Oxford University Press.

31. U.S. Congress, Joint Economic Committee, Subcommittee on Education and Health. (1989). *Medical alert, A staff report summarizing the hearings on health care in America.* Washington, DC: Institute of Medicine, National Academy Press.

32. U.S. Congress, Joint Economic Committee, Subcommittee on Education and Health. (1989). *A staff report summarizing the hearings on the future of health care in America.* Washington, DC: Institute of Medicine.

33. Wallerstein, N., & Bernstein, E. (1988, Winter). Empowerment education: Freire's ideas adapted to health education. *Health Education Quarterly, 15,* 379–394.
34. Young, S. T. (1992, May 25). Urban blacks: A study in alienation. *Philadelphia Inquirer,* p. A14.

CHAPTER EIGHT

Nursing and the Managed Care Marketplace

Claire M. Fagin and Leah F. Binder

The Clinton Administration's ambitious attempt to restructure the nation's health care delivery system failed in Congress. Yet the progress of reorganization of health care delivery continues unabated, and appears to be accelerating at state and national levels, notwithstanding the federal government's inability to reach consensus and take a leading role on how it should occur. The central characteristic of this reorganization is the growth of private sector managed care networks. The growth of managed care brings opportunity and threat for both the nursing profession and the public.

In the new managed delivery settings, roles have changed. Physicians are no longer unquestioned authorities; administrators are involved in clinical decisionmaking; and consumers are expected to be active proponents—not passive recipients—of quality care. As advocates, leaders, and educators, nurses will be valuable allies for

Note: This was originally published in Joanne McCloskey and Helen Grace, *Current Issues in Nursing*, Mosby, St. Louis, 1996, under the title "Dangerous Liaisons: Nursing, Consumers and the Managed Care Marketplace." It is reprinted here with permission.

consumers making the transition to managed environments. This chapter will examine the managed care phenomenon and its implications for nurses and consumers of care. We will argue that consumers need to develop partnerships with nurses, and that nurses should be taking an active leadership role in helping to evaluate the current organizational "reforms" so as to ensure quality and safety of care.

MANAGED CARE

Managed care networks come in numerous forms, including Preferred Provider Organizations (PPOs), Health Maintenance Organizations, coordinated care arrangements, and other so-called integrated systems. All managed care organizations share some fundamental characteristics. They limit the range of providers available to members, and they monitor and sometimes restrict the health services enrolled members are permitted to utilize. Unlike traditional fee-for-service plans that reimburse providers for each patient visit, managed care arrangements often pay providers a set ("capitated") monthly rate for each patient assigned to them, regardless of how often the patient visits if at all. Thus in managed care the provider has a financial incentive to provide the least quantity of services necessary to preserve the patient's health. Many managed care arrangements require members to affiliate with a case manager and/ or primary care provider, who may serve as a gatekeeper referring patients to specialists and other services as needed. As a result of the financial incentives and policies to coordinate care and monitor patients' utilization of services, most managed care networks are able to offer cost savings to members (Congressional Budget Office, 1994).

Increasing numbers of Americans are enrolling in managed care. As of 1994 47 million Americans were enrolled in health maintenance organizations, while another 50 million are members of preferred provider organizations (HIAA, 1995). Even traditional fee-for-service arrangements have begun to implement a process borrowed from managed care called "utilization review," in which insurance companies and not providers have the final say on the services enrollees utilize. Almost all employees covered by employer-based private insurance are now subject to some form of utilization review (Congressional Budget Office, 1992).

Since the early 1990's, managed care arrangements have grown very rapidly in the private sector and have become increasingly the mode of choice in the public sector. Overall, the jury is still out on whether managed care arrangements enhance the quality of care. The literature is contradictory on managed care's impact on the number of provider visits per patient (i.e., Hurley, Freund, and Paul, 1993, and Yhohlen et al., 1990), but there is strong evidence that managed care enrollees are far less likely than people in other kinds of plans to visit specialists (Rowland et al., 1995, p. 16). There is a decline in emergency room use and some evidence of declines in overall hospitalization (Rowland et al., 1995, p. 16). To date, studies have not found evidence that managed care improves utilization of preventive services. Among Medicaid participants, managed care has not improved the number of prenatal visits, immunizations, and well-child visits (Rowland et al., 1995, p. 17). These findings are particularly disappointing for this most vulnerable population.

There have been incidences of abuse and fraud in managed care organizations, particularly those serving Medicaid participants. A series of investigative pieces in a Florida newspaper gained national attention when it unveiled a host of abuses in several HMOs that enrolled Medicaid participants. Problems cited included neglectful providers allowing illness to go undetected and untreated; administrative costs exceeding 50% and in some cases 60% of revenues; fraudulent marketing techniques; and in one case the employment of a convicted felon as chief executive officer (Schulte, F., & J. Bergal, 1994). Questions about managed care organizations with publicly funded enrollees prompted the Health Care Financing Administration to adopt new regulations to curb abuses (*Managed Medicare & Medicaid News*, 1995, p. 1). More recently, reports from New York State and City indicate that " . . . sweeping efforts to turn over health care for Medicaid recipients to private managed care companies had been moving too quickly with too little government oversight" (The New York Times, August 28, 1995).

The current form of the managed care industry is dominated by the private sector. The combination of fiscal responsibility to share holders and government payors, with the focus on cost *containment* (rather than cost effectiveness) and control over patient utilization

of care, has some risk potential. Recognition of the deficits in evaluation of managed care practice suggests that regulation and oversight
may be important to ensure that quality of care is not sacrificed to
profit considerations. Discussions and actions with regard to such
regulation are underway in several States (e.g., New Jersey, Maryland).

Despite the foregoing cautionary notes, we believe that managed
care organizations ultimately offer the most promising solution to the
nation's health care problems. As the population ages, accelerating
health costs necessitate better coordination of care for Americans.
Fee for service arrangements, in which providers are financially reimbursed for every service provided, offer patients wide choices and
for those workers who have generous health benefit plans it is natural
that these arrangements are the package of choice. However, there
is little evidence that in the aggregate, these expensive packages of
benefits are any more effective than managed care at assuring quality
of care.

THE NURSING MODEL OF CARE

The "philosophy" undergirding managed care is, in many respects,
consonant with the nursing model of care. Like nursing, managed
care philosophy emphasizes the "whole patient," coordination of
care, and prevention and primary care. Most managed care arrangements monitor and some disclose data on quality and cost-effectiveness of providers and services; and most emphasize collaboration
between health professionals (Appleby, 1995, p. 26).

The convergence of the managed care philosophy with the professional belief system of nursing might suggest nursing's moment has
arrived. We believe that this is indeed the case. However, vast changes
in hospitals caused by reduction both in patient stay and in hospital
usage, are having severe effects on nurses. More than two thirds of
nurses work in hospitals, thus radical reductions in the numbers of
hospital beds have to have a direct impact on nursing staff. In addition, hospitals are attempting to lower costs in ways which may prove
noxious to both nurses and patients by layoffs of nurses irrespective
of patient need, reducing nurse-patient ratios at many delivery settings, and reclassification of nursing responsibilities into more am-

biguous categories of patient services (Manthey, 1995). In short, despite the centrality of nursing philosophy to the emerging managed delivery systems, nurses themselves appear increasingly marginalized.

The fact that hospitals have become increasingly reliant on managed care organizations to supply patients does not militate against excellent quality nursing care. The fact that the financial incentives under managed care to minimize the amount of care provided result in efforts to reduce per-patient costs does not militate against excellent quality nursing care. Rather, these circumstances present opportunities to nurses to develop and articulate to hospital management and to the public strong patient care systems which are cost effective and not harmful to the patient. Nurse specialist transitional care, for example, helps counter the fragmentation of care that many consumers experience as they navigate among different providers, treatments, and settings. Nurse-managed, hospital based programs to provide transitional care for patients diagnosed with cancer, for perinatal care of mother and infant, for the frail elderly, for patients with AIDS and for many other populations have been shown to be extremely effective. Study after study reinforces the value of nurses in enhancing quality and cost-effectiveness. A recent study by Linda Aiken and others found a significant correlation between the organization of nursing and mortality rates at the hospital studied (Aiken et al., 1994). A much earlier study by Draper found that strong collaboration between registered nurses and physicians resulted in 58% more patients surviving than expected (Draper, 1987). Research has shown mortality rates lower in hospitals with higher nurse-patient ratios (Hartz, Krakauer, Kuhn, 1989), and a correlation between levels of nursing and quality of patient care (Carter, Mills, & Homan, 1987; Krakauer, Bailey, & Skellan, 1992).

One model of the Advanced Practice Nurse (APN) is a consumer oriented cost effective solution for hospitals. This model, a hospital based tertiary care practitioner (TNP), blends the nurse practitioner role with the clinical nurse specialist role (Keane & Richmond, 1993).

The development of the APN was stimulated by two parallel forces: one, nursing's recognition that care should be offered by the most cost-effective providers familiar with therapeutic options in the most appropriate setting, and two, the decrease in the size of medical specialty residency programs resulting from an excess number of physician specialists in the United States. The tertiary care nurse practitioner programs are designed to provide care to complex hospitalized patients with specialized needs. These nurses have an "in-depth knowledge of the specialty's health problems and the technology used, coupled with the generalist approach reflecting nursing's holistic view of the individual . . . " (Keane & Richmond, 1993).

An excellent example of the implementation of the TNP role occurs at the Columbia-Presbyterian Medical Center in Manhattan. On selected units of the hospital TNPs do initial assessments, write admission orders, work with attending physicians to review plans of care, and work with the nursing staff to interpret clinical information and explain the rationale for treatment plans. Henry Silver, a pioneer in the nurse practitioner movement, predicted and recommended the development of a hospital based nurse practitioner role in an article published in 1988 (Silver & McAtee, 1988). "They would perform many functions and provide many services given by first-year residents in teaching hospitals."

However, despite the proven effective contributions of nurses in these roles and others, and the obvious compatibility of nursing's professional identity with the goals and priorities of managed care, nurses appear increasingly marginalized within managed care organizations, and even more serious, are often excluded from the process of planning change in organization of hospital patient care. Since nursing care is *the* essential ingredient of the patient's hospitalization, the lack of involvement of nurses in planning patient oriented change is incomprehensible.

The message that nursing is incidental and not integral to the goal of good patient care services appears to have been heard. The recent trends in hospitals mentioned above—downsizing nursing staff independent of downsizing the patient population, replacement of nurses with unlicensed personnel, eliminating mention of nursing credentials in identification of staff, increased reports of resignations or removals of directors of nursing, and eliminations of positions for clinical nurse specialists, are clear signs of intent to minimize professional nursing roles in our hospitals.

Hospitals are not the only delivery settings discounting nursing resources. Although primary care and case management are central to the managed care model and physician shortages are frequently cited, nurses' ability to provide cost-effective primary care is also being compromised (i.e., Clark, 1995, p. 19). For instance, in many states implementing Medicaid managed care, waivers override federal directives requiring direct reimbursement for certain advanced nurse providers to require physician-only case management (Keepnews, 1995, p. 16).

Even as the role and experience of nurses are marginalized, the responsibilities traditionally attributed to nurses are being extolled as central to the delivery of care. Health policy expert Stephen Shortell from the Kellogg School of Management at Northwestern University put it this way: "We need to take responsibility for more of the whole process of patient care. That is what total quality management is all about. We need more cross-training, more multi-disciplinary teams, better information systems, and new ways to treat the "entire" patient" (Shortell, 1995, p. 28). This line could have come from any nursing textbook or nursing research journal from ten or twenty years ago. Yet as the delivery system moves to embrace this model, it frequently reinvents the wheel instead of turning to the providers with the proven experience to implement it: Nurses.

What accounts for the paradox that nurses are devalued while the emerging model of health care delivery replicates the nursing model of care? At least one explanation lies in the classic conundrum of the nursing profession: Nurses control their own education but not their practice. Thus nursing has never been able to adequately reinforce a wholly independent professional identity in the practice setting. First stated by Flexner in 1915, a short list of characteristics of independent professions would include " . . . power to control the terms, conditions, and contents of work" (Friedson, 1977). The power to control one's work has been the principal differentiation between the way medicine and nursing have progressed, and organized their systems.

Two additional explanations seem as cogent. First, nurses' writings are generally not read by anyone but nurses. Thus the teaching that nurses do with regard to their models of care reaches nurses but not the public, professional or otherwise. Second, when nurses bring ·up the fact that the newer organizations or ideas were discussed and taught by nurses years ago, their comments are often dismissed by words or in non-verbal behavior. After all what powerful group wishes to hear a group without power say it has invented what they are taking credit for?

Without full and independent control over the practice of nursing, nurses are a group without direct power and nursing can appear to be a wholly dependent component of the practice setting. Managed care reformers may then identify nurses as hospital representatives, part and parcel of the delivery setting, instead of independently credentialed professionals with a set of coherent values and goals. The tendency to see nursing as part of the old ways may be compounded by the fact many of the changemakers are not providers themselves, but business executives and policymakers with little experience in direct patient care and unfamiliar with the role of nurses and the needs of patients.

COLLABORATIONS THAT WORK

Not all managed care organizations overlook nursing expertise and resources. We are seeing increasing interest in nurse practitioners in managed care organizations and other innovative practice settings that are community based.

There have also been signs that managed care organizations are employing more nurses as direct primary care providers and/or case managers. There are two kinds of case manager roles advanced nurse providers are found in. One type utilizes APNs to deliver and manage care of various populations such as the chronically mentally ill, medically fragile patients, patients with AIDS, and clients with preventive or maintenance needs. The APNs coordinate the care of these clients and manage their entry into other parts of the health care system. Others use the term casemanager to mean gatekeeper roles without direct care responsibilities. These call upon the nurse to make decisions about the kind of care, the length of the treatment, and the appropriateness of care.

Furthermore, the potential for nursing leadership in collaboration with managed care organizations has never been as dramatic. There are at least 300 nurse managed health centers such as community clinics nationwide, many affiliated with schools of nursing and other institutions (Barger & Rosenfeld, 1993; Hothaus, 1993). In South Carolina, a Family Health Center managed by a nurse practitioner developed as a community alternative to inappropriate use of the Emergency Room. In a six month period the NPs had seen almost

5000 clients. In Arizona, a nurse managed center is projecting cost savings of $500,000 in its first year, based on fewer inpatient days and emergency room visits for 18,500 enrollees. The program utilizes APNs to provide both direct care and integrated case management to patients with multisystem, chronic diseases, requiring extensive health care interventions; the program tends to focus on patients with limited socioeconomic and familial/cultural resources (Barger & Rosenfeld, 1993).

Among the many nurse managed centers of the University of Pennsylvania School of Nursing, the West Philadelphia Community Health Corner is an interesting model. Started by a faculty member and students from the University of Pennsylvania Division of Pediatric Nursing with strong cooperation from neighborhood groups, the Corner addresses the specific health needs of the community in its neighborhood setting. It offers services to children and adolescents. Immunization services, physicals, screening, walk-in pregnancy testing, birth control advice, STD testing, driver's license and sport physicals. The nurses are reimbursed directly for their services through federal and state programs.

Other current nurse managed centers at Penn include a day care hospital, and a recreation center based family health care service. Additional centers are being developed at Penn and at other University schools of nursing in the United States.

School and community center clinics, expanded home health visits, and work site health programs have mushroomed in recent years and utilize nurse practitioners almost exclusively. The settings may differ one from the other in the type of services and the background of the nurse provider. All stress prevention and maintenance of health give opportunities for innovation on the part of nurse leaders. Many of them involve the community in planning and monitoring services. The notion of marketing prevention and risk reduction in vulnerable populations is implicitly or explicitly part of many nursing centers.

NURSING LEADERSHIP

The nursing profession is experiencing chaos in the current downsizing. We believe that major adjustments are needed in relation to the size of the nursing student population and where they are being educated. It has become clear in recent years that in a greatly reduced nursing marketplace the Associate Degree Nurse will not have the opportunities that have been present in the health field during a time of expansion and nursing shortage. The current chaos should not get in the way of nursing's recognition of the potential of a managed care system for patients and for the nursing profession, if quality is monitored and assured. Nursing's proven expertise and cost-effectiveness suggest the future can be bright for nursing's involvement in the delivery systems of the future. Yet there is opposite potential as well. If nurses are so preoccupied with the current problems they may be unable to collaborate aggressively to help develop the best future models. Unless nurses assert the authority and knowledge base of the profession it is possible that change will soar forward without them.

While we have argued that the nursing model of care coincides with the philosophy of managed care organizations, the two philosophies differ in one crucial respect. Nursing has no profit motive, while most managed care organizations—whether simply to survive or for the accumulation of wealth—are guided in large part by the demands of the dollar. Certainly nurses have enjoyed the more recent fair earnings and have deserved to be paid equitable salaries. However, their primary focus is on patient care. Thus occasionally nurses may diverge from their managed care colleagues when they seek to esteem the quality of patient care over and above the cost of that care. Often enough, quality and cost-effectiveness go hand in hand, such as in gatekeeping functions that help patients avoid unnecessary and dangerous procedures. But when they do not, nurses must remain as critical patient advocates.

Unless nurses assert the value of nursing as a voice for cost effective, quality care and a profession with ideals compatible to managed care, the contributions of nurses and the profession will be at risk and the safety and well-being of patients will be compromised. There are immediate, sometimes severe, consequences to patients when nursing leadership is devalued, when per-patient nursing staff levels are lowered, when inadequately trained workers are placed at the bedside, and when nursing's experience and knowledge are excluded from provider collaborations, planning, and coordinated care.

Nurse educators have an obligation to prepare nursing students for the world of managed care, including both clinical aspects and issues of financing and administration. But concurrently, nurse educators need to understand the techniques of community organization and leadership and the importance of building partnerships and coalitions with the public. These concomitant and sometimes conflictual learnings are crucial if nurses believe they can effect quality care. Providers without an understanding of the business of managed care are at a distinct disadvantage in the new cost-dominated delivery systems. Providers without an understanding of the role of the active consumer will be equally disadvantaged. Nurse researchers should reflect how their research can apply to managed care and develop proposals to investigate and uncover best practices. Despite its prevalence, managed care is in many respects in its infancy, when new research and data can offer pioneering new directions with the potential to shape health care reform. It is interesting, for example, that managed care has been largely unable to improve certain kinds of preventive care such as prenatal visits. Can nurse researchers learn how to improve the record? We think so.

No group of professionals better understands the philosophy of managed care and how to implement it than nurses. John Gardner's views (1964) on the tasks of leadership describe what leaders must do and offer a blueprint for nurses to consider in their daily work:

1. Envisioning goals
2. Affirming Values
3. Motivating
4. Managing
   —Planning and priority setting
   —Organizing and institution building
   —Keeping the system functioning
   —Agenda setting and decisionmaking
   —Exercising political judgment
5. Achieving workable unity
6. Explaining
7. Serving as a symbol
8. Representing the group
9. Renewing

Nurses must take leadership to preserve the vision, goals, values, and symbols of good health care that brought them to the health care system. Nurses should not quietly step aside to give others an exclusive forum to educate the public and set direction on issues like preventive care and coordination of care that are the lifeblood of nursing experience and knowledge. By upholding the autonomy and professionalism of the nursing role—recognizing that autonomy is not lost in partnership with consumers—and asserting that health care quality is the raison d'être for professionalism, nurses have the opportunity as never before to help set the direction for and implement positive health care reform.

REFERENCES

Aiken, L., Smith, H., & Lake, E. (1994). Lower Medicare mortality among a set of hospitals known for good nursing care. *Medical Care, 32*(8).

Alan Guttmacher Institute. (1995). Special analysis: How family planning services fare under state bids to restructure Medicaid. *State Reproductive Health Monitor, 6*(2), p. 3.

American Nurse. (1995). Survey finds loss of RNs jeopardizes patient safety. Jan/Feb, 1.

Appleby, C. (1995). The measure of medical services. *Hospitals & Health Networks, June 20,* 26.

Barger, S., & Rosenfeld, P. (1993). Models in community health care: Findings from a national study of community nursing centers. *Nursing & Health Care, 14*(8), 426–431.

Beyers, M. (1995). The consequences of change. *Nursing Management, 26*(5), 22.

Clark, C. S. (1995). Defining primary care. *Healthcare Financial Management,* January, 19.

Congressional Budget Office. (1994). *Effects of Managed Care: An Update.* Washington, DC: CBO.

Congressional Budget Office. (1994). *Effects of Managed Care: An Update.* CBO Memorandum, Washington, DC: CBO, March.

Draper, E. A. (1987). Effects of nurse/physician collaboration and nursing standards on ICU patient outcomes. 1(4), 2–8.

Fagin, C. M., & Binder, L. F. (1994). Nursing and consumerism: How can we get decision making closer to the consumer? In *Current Issues in Nursing.* Mosby, St. Louis. pp. 450–459.

Fisher, I., & Fein, E. B. (1995). Forced Marriage of Medicaid and Medicare Hits Snags, *The New York Times*, August 28.

Friedson, E. (1977). The future of professionalization. In J. W. Gardner (Ed.), *Self Renewal*. New York: Perennial Library.

HIAA. (1995). *Source Book of Health Insurance Data 1994*. Washington, DC: Health Insurance Association of America.

Health Care Financing Administration, Office of Managed Care. (1994). *Medicaid Managed Care Enrollment Report Summary statistics as of June 30, 1994*. Washington, DC: U.S. Dept. of Health & Human Services.

Hothaus, R. (1993). Nurse-managed health care: An ongoing tradition. *Nurse Practitioner Forum*, 4(3), 128–132.

Hurley, R., Freund, D., & Paul, J. (1993). *Managed care in Medicaid: Lessons for policy and program design*. Ann Arbor, MI: Heath Administration Press.

Keepnews, D. (1995). State Medicaid waivers: Issues for nurses. *American Nurse*, Apr/May, 16.

Managed Medicare & Medicaid News. (1995). GAO Questions HCFA vigilance against quality violations by Medicare risk contract HMOs, 24(31), 1.

Manthey, M. (1995). Marie Manthey interviews Norma Lang. *Creative Nursing, March/April*, 7.

Morgan, N. (1995). Health-care gurus view San Diego as model. *The San Diego Union-Tribune*, Jan. 15.

Rowland, D., Rosenbaum, S., Simon, L., & Chait, E. (1995). *Medicaid and Managed Care: Lessons from the Literature*. Washington, DC: The Henry J. Kaiser Family Foundation.

Schulte, F., & Bergal, J. (1994). Florida's Medicaid HMO's: Profits From Pain. *Sun Sentinel*, Dec. 11–15.

Shortell, S. M. (1995). The Future of Integrated Systems. *Health Care Financial Management*, *24*, January, 28.

Silver, H. K., & McAtee, P. (1988). Should nurses substitute for House staff? *American Journal of Nursing*, 1671–1673.

CHAPTER NINE

The Abandonment of the Patient: The Impact of For-Profit Health Care

Claire M. Fagin and Suzanne Gordon

The mid to late 1990s have brought momentous issues to those of us who have devoted our lives to ensuring quality care to patients and families. The pendulum has swung from the "never mind the cost" philosophy of two decades ago to the bottom line philosophy of today. Health care providers, long sheltered by 3rd party cost reimbursement policies are now facing the spectre of cost competition. The anticipated reductions in Medicare and Medicaid benefits will exacerbate the scramble to devise strategies to compete. The influence of for-profit managed care and home health care companies is driving the not for profits out of the market or causing them to bring down costs in order to stay in business.

We link the abandonment of the patient to the corporatization of health care. The original concept of managed care aimed to help the patient negotiate the increasingly complex world of health care and change the focus of care to prevention, coordination of services, and the like. Managed care is now more and more likely to mean

Note: A version of this chapter was published as the last chapter of *Abandonment of the Patient: The Impact of Profit-Driven Health Care on the Public,* by E. D. Baer, C. Fagin, and S. Gordon. New York: Springer Publishing, 1996.

cost control and cost reduction. Overloaded and undertrained care givers, early discharge from hospitals to inadequate home care, less choice, more out of pocket cost, and reduced access to health care. All this and the direct effect of a cap on Medicare and Medicaid is yet to be felt.

Every health care system must manage care, indeed, must ration care. But the operative word, principle and philosophy must be *care*, not *profit*. We believe, with many others that managed care organizations can ultimately offer the most promising solution to the nation's health care problems. Coordination of care has always been a problem in traditional, acute care focused medicine. Too much care—that is, unnecessary or inappropriate care—not only has cost money but has made patients vulnerable to harmful side effects. As the population ages, the needs of patients coupled with accelerating health costs necessitate a system of care which provides better coordination, less fragmentation, awareness of the complete health record, preventive services, and education. While many of us might personally prefer fee for service arrangements which offer us wide choices paid for by generous health benefit plans, there is little evidence that in the aggregate, these expensive packages of benefits are any more effective than appropriately managed care at assuring quality of care.

But there is the rub: What is appropriately managed care? No system changing as fast as health care delivery can be all good, or all safe, or all of even quality. How is the consumer to have any idea of what to look for or how to evaluate what they are getting without a regular source of information and support and without being able to maintain their trust in their health care providers and the institutions that have merited their respect for almost a century.

It is clear that we and many of our colleagues are skeptical about the marketplace invasion of health care. We are deeply concerned because we do not believe that industrial models of care and treatment should be applied to the sick and vulnerable—or to the healthy who, after all, use the health care system because they fear sickness and vulnerability.

Despite its prevalence, managed care is in many respects in its infancy, when new research and data can offer pioneering new directions with the potential to shape health care reform. We need our clinical researchers to tell us what evaluations are occurring with regard to rapid changes of restructuring and shifting of modalities for health care delivery.

We need clinical researchers to investigate and uncover best practices. We need to know about the post-hospital experiences of patients who do not have expert care. We need to know the steps being taken to adapt the services of most managed care organizations to the older or poorer, and often less healthy populations they are currently seeking to attract.

If the marketplace believes that competition is the solution to the health care crisis of this nation, then it must create a system that competes on quality. But that is not what we have today. If the HMO and insurer's real customer is the employer who purchases health care, not the employee who uses it, then there is no competition in health care. If the users of health care services do not have freedom of choice of provider, hospital, nursing home, subacute facility, home care agency, then there is no competition in health care. Let's be truthful in our discussion. How can there be competition in health care when the majority of employers who offer health benefits offer no choice of health care plan? How can we claim we are delivering genuine health care in a competitive system when employees who lose faith in an HMO, physician, or hospital are imprisoned in the very institutions they have come to distrust?

Today patient care is being redefined almost entirely in market terms, where cost rather than care has the highest priority. Those governing our health care system advertise quality but, in reality, profit from the healthy and lose money from caring for the sick.

As we learn in increasingly frequent news reports, the savings corporate managed care has wrested from the health care system are not being redirected toward the long overdue effort to insure the uninsured. Savings are not even being directed to enhancing the delivery of care to those with health insurance. Nor are savings being directed to education and research.

One HMO executive recently expressed his delight to see that the industrial revolution had finally penetrated the health care delivery system. Under HMO direction, he said, physicians would be turned into sophisticated machine tools programmed to deliver the care that his and other managed care companies deem appropriate. Do we really want a health care system to turn patients into predictable units of production and that transforms nurses, and physicians into assembly-line workers or supervisors? Or do we want a health care system that recognizes that illness is the ultimate unpredictable human event and that responds to the need for flexible, individualized models of care delivery?

Today, HMOs insurers and hospitals are developing standards of care, algorithms, and critical paths that determine patients fates but which are shielded from patient or public scrutiny. In their public pronouncements, health plans insist that any guidelines or standards of care are applied flexibly and are tailored to each patient's needs. We know, however, that clinicians who deviate from practice rules are penalized and that financial incentives are the name of the game for holding down medical expenses.

In December 1995, the Center for Health Care Rights in Los Angeles released a 250 page study entitled Consumer Protection in State HMO Laws. Volume 1: Analysis and Recommendations.

The study highlighted serious concerns about marketing, lack of open enrollment, and contract cancellation periods. They are worried about grievance procedures, accountability, HMO lock-in provisions, referral and utilization control systems or delays, and restricted access to care. The study's exhaustive review of state statutes reveals that, "Most states do not provide adequate protections for HMO enrollees. In every area of consumer HMO law, but especially in the areas of access, quality of care, grievance procedures, the collection, analysis and release of quality care data, and the provision of HMO information to enrollees and the public, the study found that critical legal and regulatory issues were not addressed."

Also in late 1995, the National Health Council issued a publication which lists their recommendations for consumers in examining managed care options, and during the same time period, Citizen Action and the Consumers Union released "The Managed Care Consumers' Bill of Rights." Their list of 10 fundamental rights are: access, choice, comprehensive benefits, affordability, quality, appeals, representation, and enforcement. We will expand on several of these below. But the agreement we have with these groups holds both bad news and good news. The bad news is that all these groups are gravely worried about all of the areas our speakers have spoken about today. The good news is that we are part of a growing group of consumer advocates whose actions have the potential to help mold the changing scene.

We believe there is a list of requirements that must be considered as we examine managed care and any other care system offered to the public. An overarching requirement for the survival of patients and the survival of our institutions is the assurance of a "safety net" which would impose and fund minimum standards. It is clear that this is not on the horizon at this time. If we are to protect, rather than abandon patients, choice, quality, accountability, and public disclosure should be non-negotiable.

All recent reports agree on the importance of choice. Americans, like Europeans and Canadians must have some choice of health care provider, hospital, nursing home, home care agency. Health care choices must, moreover, include preventive and counseling services, alternatives to hospitalization such as home care, birthing centers, hospice services in the home, residential hospices, and in-patient palliative care units.

We must rigorously debunk the ludicrous notion that people who can switch HMOs once a year do—in fact have a choice. If a person joins a health care plan in January, is diagnosed with pancreatic cancer in March, discovers that he does not trust his doctor, hospital, and health care plan, it is hardly of consolation to learn he or she can switch plans ten months later, after he may have died.

Second—quality: All of us are concerned about the erosion of quality of care. The Institute of Medicine (1990)[1] has defined quality as the degree to which health services for individuals and populations increase the likelihood of desired health outcomes. . . . Quality is composed of various factors. Among them are core benefits offered, the expertise of practitioners, time spent with patients, appropriate care given in the right place, trust, and access to care.

Patients have a right to caregivers who have been educated and licensed because they have mastered the art and science of delivering care. Yet today, patients are increasingly denied access to expert caregivers. Recent assessments of the oversupply of physicians and nurses are based on a variety of factors, some predicted for years and others based on the expected employment changes affecting physician specialists and nurses, produced by managed care. This linkage is unfortunate. In many institutions currently, we are seeing an artificially induced shortage of *nursing* where care resembles the early 80s when there was a real shortage of *nurses.*

Time is another element that is critical to the delivery of quality health care. Health professionals cannot deliver adequate health care services if they have no time to get to know their patients, or deliver those services. Yet, in the hospital, office, and home, practitioners and patients are being denied needed time. For example, at Kaiser in Northern California, family practice physicians now carry patient panels of 2400 to 2700 patients. That is 500 to 800 more patients than are on the panel of the British GPs—the most harried generalists in the industrialized world. It is estimated that this patient load will allow for about five minutes per patient-doctor encounter.

Quality of care also means appropriate care given in the right place. We need standards for the combination of hospital stay and home care. Today, the U.S. has the shortest length of hospital stay of any nation in the industrialized world. Genuine health care does not demand endless, unnecessary hospital stays. But it does demand that length of stay be determined by the doctor, nurse, and patient together. What determines length of stay should be the stability of the patient's condition, the safety of the home or community environment, and the quality of the caregiving available outside of the hospital.

Studies conducted at the University of Pennsylvania by Dr. Dorothy Brooten and others have confirmed the kind of excellent outcomes that are achieved when home care is delivered and monitored by advanced practice nurses.[2] Indeed, clinical expertise is even more critical in the home than in the hospital. In the hospital, a novice or inexperienced worker has at least some hope of finding an expert who can fill in the gaps of their knowledge. In the home, both patient and caregiver are on their own. To have high quality care in the home, expertise is essential.

But today more and more patients are being sent home too quickly. Once at home, care provided is very short term and the caregivers are, more and more, untrained workers. These personnel may be asked to give enemas, insulin shots, change sterile dressings, and hook up complicated machines to name only a few of the so-called tasks they are assigned.[2]

Very quickly, care is assigned to inexperienced family members— most of them women. These family members are further abandoned by a society that demands that they take time from work—or sacrifice their jobs entirely—to provide the kind of care that used to be provided in the hospital or in nursing homes. Time must be a focus of our attention as we advocate for the patient.

Trust is also a non-negotiable of quality care. But that trust is being undermined by the kind of economic blackmail that threatens professionals who try to protect quality care or journalists whose employers are concerned about losing advertising revenues or the pernicious economic incentives that reward doctors and administrators for denying needed care. As we are learning daily, physician reimbursement is explicitly linked to the denial of tests, procedures, specialist consultations, and hospital days to patients who need them. Both New Jersey and New York are revamping HMO regulations to uncover these practices.

When caregivers are encouraged to view the sick as a burden, as the "medical loss ratio" then one can only conclude that care is being managed right out of health care.

Quality health care also demands that patients have access to services when they need them. Instead, the frantic effort to contain costs has turned into an exercise of corporate gamesmanship. Consider the extraordinary phenomenon of the retrospective denial of emergency room services. A patient experiences crushing chest pain. Fearful that he is having a heart attack, he rushes to the ER. He is worked up and it is discovered that he is not having a heart attack but rather a bad attack of gastritis. That is the good news. The bad news is his insurance plan refuses to pay for this medical work-up because he did not have a heart attack. One wonders about the fevered imaginations of those who think up these ideas. But we must be mindful of their result. Patients will fear making a visit to the emergency room because they cannot predict the financial result. We are thus asking of them the impossible, and the unacceptable— that they diagnose their own complex medical conditions.

Third on our list of non-negotiables is accountability. Today, more and more patients are being asked to sign away their rights to sue an HMO for malpractice and doctors are being asked to sign away their right to hold HMOs accountable for the results of policies doctors are asked to enforce. Where is the accountability in such a system? As the new health care system is zooming to incorporate itself and all of us, it is crucial that we know about the Review and Regulatory Mechanisms governing it. What are they, who do they represent, are clinicians and patients part of the process?

The fourth non-negotiable in the evolving system must be public disclosure, which includes free access to information for patients and providers. Patients and families must have access to information that will allow them to make informed choices. We must pressure for federal, state, and local requirements for public accounting. Granted, this is a complex process but crucial if choice is to have any meaning. Such accounting should include information of the clinical guidelines that are used, and the professional oversight of these guidelines. We ought to know how much of every dollar is spent on clinical personnel, administrative personnel, and research, education, indigent care, and overhead. Further, we need information about appeals processes, grievances filed, and results.

At this time most managed care arrangements monitor, but only some disclose, data on quality and cost-effectiveness of providers and services.[3] We do know something about overhead though. The very successful managed care companies report an overhead of close to 30% as compared with Medicare which spent 1.74% in 1995 and Medicaid which spent 4.41%.[4]

Finally, we need to remind ourselves that we cannot think of quality of care while allowing the number of uninsured and underinsured Americans to rise. We must instead extend coverage to all. The fact that the U.S. spends more than a trillion dollars on health care a year—more than any other nation in the world—yet has rationed 41 million people right out of the health care system is totally unacceptable. To talk about universal coverage at this time sounds like pie in the sky. Oddly, I believe that in the next five to seven years it will be seen as a necessity, rather than an aspect of altruism. There will be no way for hospitals to manage to care for the indigent, for the uninsured middle class, to educate physicians, to participate in education of all health care providers, without a concept of universality in health care coverage. Cost shifting is at least moribund if not dead.

Many strategies for addressing the health care crisis have been discussed this afternoon. It seems to me that these strategies have three main thrusts: Publicity, Political Action, and Coalition Building.

Publicity—Nurses are part of a larger scene to publicize the abandonment of the patient in America. Voices, stories, phone calls, and letters to the media are crucial. We need these stories, particularly from patients and families of patients to get a public airing. We need to find ways to penetrate the wall of denial and economic blackmail that conceals the facts of what is happening in health and illness care today.

Political Action—Legislative representatives have responded to pressures from professional and consumer organizations about their concerns. While not yet passing a bill on patients' rights there is a great deal of discussion about this and other issues relating to managed care and the uninsured. Action on the State level is ongoing and bills have been passed in many states to provide more consumer protection, curtail the denial of emergency room services, prolong the possibility of hospitalizations in certain instances, prevent incentive programs for physicians who deny services and the like. Health care is again emerging on the public's agenda as a top priority for change. Clearly, part of any legislative agenda for change must include whistle blower protection for those employees who speak out to protect the patient and to ban the kinds of perverse gag orders and financial incentives that explicitly pit physicians against their patients.

Coalition Building—We need coalitions of health professional, hospital, and consumer groups to lobby at every governmental level and to work together to publicize the problems they see. Surely this is an area where all these groups should find common ground. Certainly no health professional brought up on the concepts of altruism and accountability wants to be forced to compete by reducing the quality of health care.

Publicity, political action, and coalition building can become part and parcel of our direct patient care roles as we help our patients advocate for themselves with their own doctors, hospitals and HMOs and in the political arena. When we hear patients, friends, family members, and neighbors complain of eroding quality care, we must urge them to call their political representatives, write and complain to state boards of health and insurance and the chairpeople of their state legislature's health committee and the media. Those of us who are patients or represent groups of patients must work to educate the public and one another about our options, and the remedies available.

In our country, we have great faith in the ability of the marketplace and of competition to serve us and our loved-ones. We believe, in spite of evidence to the contrary, that the private sector is more efficient in delivering its products. Perhaps health care is the ultimate testing ground of this mythical faith in the market.

Which is why in closing, we ask that you consider the ultimate issue. When Adam Smith and those who initially developed the ideals of the marketplace and replaced the concept of divine providence with the invisible hand, even they cautioned that the marketplace should be kept in its place and should not invade what they called civil society. Today, those warnings have not been heeded and the market is being invited into the most intimate corners of our lives.

The implications of this open invitation to a market invasion of health care cannot be ignored. Market theory posits a world of disconnected, hostile, adversarial actors guided by a winner take all ethic that reduces life to a series of exercises in competitive gamesmanship. In the marketplace, we must remember, the ruling motto is caveat emptor, buyer beware. In the battles of the competitive marketplace, this corporate gamesmanship does not posit a new age win/win scenario, but the very old scenario of winner take all. Does this world view, and its ethics and mission have anything to do with the care of sick, vulnerable, aging, or dying human beings? Can we rely on corporate dominated health care to protect patients?

We think not. Which is why we believe we must together reaffirm the conviction that the health care system must care for all members of society—whether rich or poor. We must devote our efforts to keeping people healthy as long as possible but we must insist that when people get sick—as we all ultimately do—quality care is the only bottom line which we will honor.

ENDNOTES

1. Institute of Medicine. Medicare: A strategy for Quality Assurance (2 Vols.), K. N. Lohr, ed. Washington, DC: National Academy Press, 1990.
2. *The New York Times,* November 21, 1995.
3. Appleby, C. (1995). *The measure of medical services.* Hospitals & Health Networks, June 20, 26.
4. Burner, S. T., & Waldo, D. R. (1995). National Health Expenditure Projections, 1994–2005. *Health Care Financing Review, 16,* 4:221–242.

PART TWO

Preparing Future Nurses: Leadership in Education

CHAPTER TEN

Preparing Students for Leadership

Claire M. Fagin

Nursing educators in baccalaureate and higher degree programs have tried to inculcate the notion of leadership among students for much of this century. The origin of an attitude regarding "leaders" as graduates of baccalaureate programs is fairly obvious. When the baccalaureate programs received most of their students from a practicing group of nurses it was obvious that these self-selectors were indeed the potential leaders of the emerging profession. Nursing educators maintained this view of their products long after it was viable. That is, despite the fact that the majority of students in baccalaureate programs are generic students, the educators have continued to promote the view that they are being prepared for leadership. This may be interpreted by the student in ways which inhibit positive learning (and leadership) as neophytes rather than enhance the development of leadership.

Contributing to the neophyte's distorted view of herself is, I believe, the sense of unreality between her view of leadership and her actual performance. Her view of leadership may be different from

Note: This is an updated and revised version of an article that was published in *Nursing Leadership*, Vol. 2, No. 4, December 1979. The original title was "Refocus on Leadership."

the view held by the nurse educator. That is, the nurse educator may be very clear in thinking about the level of leadership to be expected from the baccalaureate-prepared neophyte. It is my belief, however, that this clarity has not been imparted to the student. Rather, the students see leadership requirements as including change of complex systems far beyond the level of their competencies. Not being able to accomplish the impossible the young nurse all too frequently undersells the possible.

Many university schools of nursing prepare a product for some idealized version of a health service delivery system. Terminal objectives of many baccalaureate programs attest to this fact. Independence; autonomy; risk-taking; accountability; cognitive skills in behavioral, physical, and social sciences; and communication skills are expected in most programs. These characteristics are not found in the majority of practicing nurses nor are they fostered in the current health delivery system.

Even when such disparities are acknowledged it is rare that experiences are built into curricula which help students understand levels of leadership, steps of change, realistic expectations about change, how to negotiate for and accept power, and other armaments for the successful management of their role transition. Rather they are told they are being prepared for a system which somehow through their leadership they must change so that it can accommodate *their* learning—change which their faculty has been unable to accomplish. The vast majority of faculty members in schools of nursing have themselves had little experience as leaders in nursing practice; thus new graduates are often exhorted to make the world better than they find it, using essentially untested ideas for change making.

Corwin[1] points out the special problems which occur when teachers are not practitioners and comments that teachers, like parents, are easily tempted to project their fantasies, ideals, and aspirations upon their students.

Everyone is victimized by this dichotomy between the real and fantasy world of health services. The consumer is losing the benefit of well-prepared, committed intelligent group of people dedicated at the start to meeting their health needs. The nurses, finding themselves unable to cope with the role conflict and lack of support in the work world, maladapt or flee from nursing altogether, or move into graduate education where later they will repeat the teaching of fantasies.

Educational programs in nursing preparing for leadership are usually said to include baccalaureate and higher degree programs. This goal on the part of the programs is compatible with the goals of the entering students. Indeed, baccalaureate graduates chose this route for career advancement and opportunities for future success.

This compatibility of goals offers educators an ideal situation for planning learning experiences. Some components necessary for this learning have been identified by others. I believe they include:

1. The recognition that levels of leadership differ at different stages of educational preparation, *maturity*, and specific interest. Clear identification in the learning experience of the level of leadership intended.
2. The ability to refocus and refine problems, regardless of level of leadership, often in the face of hostility, anxiety, or alienation.
3. The ability to articulate the problem and pose a variety of solutions.
4. The demonstration by faculty of real life solutions to real life problems.

This chapter will discuss these components of learning as they pertain to the first level of leadership only—that is, the expected leadership potential of the baccalaureate graduate. Success during this adult developmental period is essential for further growth in leadership.

The recognition that levels of leadership differ at different stages of educational preparation, maturity, and specific interest. Clear identification in the learning experience of the level of leadership intended. Baccalaureate graduates are composed of three groups: 22-year-olds who entered the program directly from high school; R.N.s from A.D. or hospital schools who may range in age from 22–?; non-nursing degree entrants usually between 25 and 40 years old. My experience indicated most graduates are between 22 and 25 years old and have a range of nonstudent nursing experience from 0–3 years.

While the nonnurse background graduate expects to practice at the beginning level for some period of time, the R.N. graduate frequently is preparing for some level of leadership.

Given the age and background of most graduates, what should be the focus of expected leadership for the first experience in nursing?

Faculty members need to clearly answer this question for themselves and be able then to communicate both the expectation and the known competencies which the graduates have to fulfill the expectation.

The neophyte baccalaureate graduate should be helped to focus her attention on two incremental steps.

1. Achieving success in nurse-patient relationship which includes:
   a. focus on the one-to-one and small group (personal and family) affecting the success of this interaction.
   b. assessing the environment as it affects above.
   c. testing personal behaviors to accomplish goals and beginning to develop sense of what works.
   d. establishing self as a "person" in work area.
2. Achieving success in small group participation and leadership which includes:
   a. meeting objectives for quality patient care by influencing others as well as by direct action on unit.
   b. interprofessional activities focusing on patient care.
   c. becoming known to patients, families, nursing personnel and members of other disciplines *on unit* as person who fulfills the learned professional nursing role and can articulate it.

To accomplish these two steps as a new graduate the nurse must have competency in: Problem solving; technical skills; interpersonal skills; knowledge of social systems and experience in assessment and manipulation of role in small groups; ability and willingness to take risks based on knowledge.

In addition to these generalized expectations, individual interests will dictate specific areas for leadership in organization work, political activities, legislative activities, etc. While each individual creates her own future in such areas the peer group support inherent in these activities should be made evident early on in educational programs.

The ability to refocus and refine problems, regardless of level of leadership, often in the face of hostility, anxiety, or alienation.

Problem-solving ability is the *sine qua non* of the activity-oriented professional. Progressive levels of knowledge gained through intellectual pursuits and experience form the data to permit problem solution at different levels of leadership. For the neophyte the problems at hand pertain to the focus for leadership described above. What frequently reduces the young nurse's effectiveness in use of this learned skill is the anxiety and impotence generated in the new position. Esther Lucille Brown (unpublished data) has commented:

> Nothing is borne in more emphatically on anyone who has attempted to study and understand the nursing profession than the realization that a large segment of the profession lives within a culture of denial: the denial of reality concerning the existence of health problems, the denial of the inherent ability and the responsibility of the profession to improve health care services; the denial even of one's own self-worth and self-importance as a professional person. So strong is this culture of denial that it not only tends to reduce its constituency to a feeling of impotence that almost precludes positive action, but it acts as a psychological barrier that must be slowly and painfully scaled by that other and smaller sector of the profession that is intent on producing change.

Yet even this small "intent on producing change" is confronting the bureaucratic structure of most health-related facilities and their special characteristics. Adherence to rules, conformity and subsequent interference with individual adaptation, depersonalization of relationships, and alienation are all seen to a more or less degree and influence the young nurse's role performance.

How then to accomplish a professional role of problem solving which by its very definition requires individual adaptations? The learnings preceding graduation must include a pseudo real life experience where students play a staff role. This experience must be accompanied by a dissection of the components of the experience using social systems theories. I have found classic articles such as Merton's "Bureaucratic Structure and Personality"[2] and Rose Laub Coser's "Alienation and the Social Structure"[3] particularly useful in this regard.

To concretely help the student assess the social system I have used the outline shown in Table 10.1.

TABLE 10.1   How to Look at Social System of Institutions

I.   *WHY*—Philosophy
    A. What is stated—where?
    B. How is it implemented?

II. *COMMUNICATION*
    A. *Channels*
       1. Verbal
          a. Formal—meetings, group individual.
             What kind?—does someone lecture or are announcements made?
             Who is involved? Who leads?
             What is the level and disciplines?
             Rounds—what is discussed?
          b. Informal—who, what, when, and where.
             Who is left out?
       2. Written
          a. Reports—About what?
             Frequency?
             To and from.
             What is required and type?
             Announcements and proclamations.
          b. Limits to Communication.
             Time.
             People don't read reports.
             Confidentiality.
             Omission of some staff.

III. *POWER STRUCTURE*
    A. What is the hierarchy—"For real."
                    actual.
                    observed.
    B. Decision making—How and at what level?
                    Concerning what?
    C. Policies—What they are?
                    How determined and how implemented?
                    Are they observed?

IV. *PROGRAM AND ROUTINES*
    A. Purpose—may vary.
    B. Type.
    C. How used?
    D. General philosophy—what are the limits?

V.   *STAFF*
    A. Roles, patterning—who, when, does what?
    B. Job description and performance.
    C. Qualifications of staff.

The ability to articulate the problem and pose a variety of solutions. As has been well established, nurses experience contradictory demands and expectations from members of their work environment. All too frequently problems with patients, co-workers, and others are felt but not clearly stated by the nurse. Making the problem manifest will accomplish several goals: If it concerns conflict with others, articulation will frequently redirect the conflict. Making the problem manifest will aid in finding solutions since others also may be concerned with the same problem and have data not available to the problem stated. Articulating the problem is inherently ego building since it is a personalizing behavior in an oftentimes depersonalizing situation. Another gain is the encouragement of consensual validation and group support.

Early on, the possible solutions available to the neophyte are limited. Through sharing, learning, testing, risking, the possibilities will increase.

Again, the learning and practice of this skill is crucial to the educational program. Important to this component of leadership and to the two preceding is what Foote and Cottrell describe as interpersonal competence.[4]

Interpersonal competence is the skill or set of abilities allowing an individual to shape the responses he gets from others. This involves correctly predicting the impact of one's own actions on the other person's definition of the situation, having a varied and large repertoire of possible lines of action and the necessary interpersonal resources to employ appropriate tactics. It is the vital characteristic in leadership.

It is clear that interpersonal competence is a developmental term. That is, given that it can be taught, it must be recognized that experience, maturity, adaptability, openness, and self-confidence will contribute to increased competence. It is an infinite quality which contributes to leadership skills at every level.

Assuming that successful resolution of the transition between student role and expectations and work role and expectations requires interpersonal competence it is necessary to define those theoretical and practical learnings which will provide the young practitioner with the resources for appropriate action.

The three components I have outlined for planning learning experiences in leadership include both cognitive learnings and interpersonal learnings. While the intended outcome must be recognized throughout the educational experience, the integration of the content in the student cannot occur until a sufficient level of technical skill has been reached. This permits the student to focus attention on the situation.

The demonstration by faculty of real-life solutions to real-life problems. It has become clear to many of us that learning opportunities for nursing students are diminished when there is absence of a practicing role model faculty. Faculties and nurses in collaborating health facilities facilitate sharing, joint practice-teaching roles, clinical demonstration, and other forms of clinical nursing models which have mutual benefit.

PROGRESSION TO SUBSEQUENT STAGES

While this chapter has dealt with leadership expectations of the baccalaureate graduate, Figure 10.1 presents a grid suggesting leadership development.

The triangle in Figure 10.1 presupposes the continuation of leadership development where each variable becomes more complex as the nurse grows in depth experience, education, and maturity.

For the first stage on there are incremental changes in the following areas:

- Problem-solving skills
- Technical skills
- Interpersonal skills
- Knowledge of social systems and competency in change skills
- Risk-taking
- Group leadership

Some of the growth occurs as a result of experience put to intellectual use; other occurs through formalized learning experiences. For the fully developed leader engaging in health policy activities credibility is enhanced by accepted "degrees," publications, organization activities, speeches, etc.

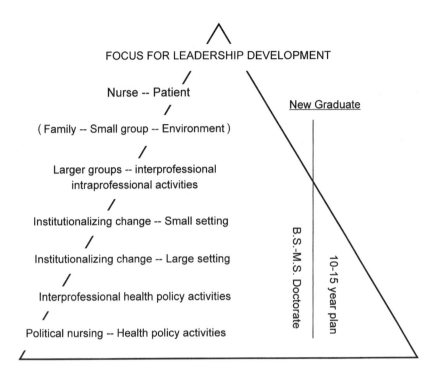

FOCUS FOR LEADERSHIP DEVELOPMENT

Nurse -- Patient

(Family -- Small group -- Environment)

Larger groups -- interprofessional
intraprofessional activities

Institutionalizing change -- Small setting

Institutionalizing change -- Large setting

Interprofessional health policy activities

Political nursing -- Health policy activities

New Graduate

B.S.-M.S. Doctorate

10-15 year plan

FIGURE 10.1

SUMMARY AND CONCLUSION

This chapter has considered leadership development and refocused on leadership expectations of the baccalaureate graduate. I commented on what I see as unrealistic goals overtly or covertly set for the neophyte. These have often mitigated against change by presenting impossible hopes or challenges which in the process of not being realized become additional areas of frustration.

Four components of leadership were examined from the standpoint of levels, competencies, and learning experiences. The fluidity of nursing permits leaders to develop optimistic clarity on the part of faculty and students will enhance this process.

ENDNOTES

1. Corwin, R. (1965). The professional employee: A study of conflict in nursing roles. In Skipper, Leonard (Eds.), *Social Interaction and Patient Care* (pp. 341–356). Philadelphia: J. B. Lippincott Co.
2. Merton, R. (1968). Bureaucratic structure and personality. In *Social theory and social structure* (pp. 249–261). Glencoe, IL: The Free Press.
3. Coser, R. L. (1963). Alienation and the social structure. In E. Friedson (Ed.), *The Hospital in Modern Society* (pp. 231–265). Glencoe, IL: The Free Press.
4. Foote, N., & Cottrell, L. (1955). *Identity and Interpersonal Competence* (pp. 41–42). Chicago: University of Chicago Press.

CHAPTER ELEVEN

An Agenda for Nursing Education

Claire M. Fagin and Joan E. Lynaugh

N ursing starts the 2000s with a radically different persona. The public at large respects nurses; nursing has become more visible for its services both in hospitals and the community; the image of submissive, oppressed women—so long held— seems to be disappearing. Almost half the public polled in 1989 believes that nurses have at least baccalaureate degrees, and, based on that belief, accepts expanded practice for nurses.[1]

The truth is, only 28.8% of registered nurses receive their basic education in baccalaureate programs and fewer than a third hold the baccalaureate degree achieved by any route.[1a] We might say we are duping the public. For this and other reasons, we must reopen the debate about preparation for entry to professional nursing practice. After providing a brief frame of reference, we propose here to reflect on the history of education and practice of nurses, discuss the contemporary scene, and raise crucial questions about the future. We

Note: This is an updated and revised version of an article that was published in *Nursing Outlook*, September/October 1972, Vol. 40, No. 5. It is reprinted here with permission. The original title was "Reaping the Rewards of Radical Change: A New Agenda for Nursing Education."

will then recommend proposals to forge a more responsive, creative nurse education system.

New nurses graduate from community colleges, 4-year colleges, university programs granting BSNs, MSNs, and doctoral degrees, and hospital programs, some of which may be degree granting. This large and unwieldy system produces impressive numbers of graduates. Though enrollments have declined, nursing schools still graduated 94,098 new RNs in 1998.[2]

The common responsibility we all share is how nurses are prepared for their work. As a practice profession, nursing can justify its existence only through the individual nurse's therapeutic effectiveness. Nurses now accept cultural authority for their own professional actions. Nurses are expected to exercise excellent clinical judgment, dispense care, and be accountable for their actions. If our clinical care "bridges" fall, we must, like structural engineers, take the blame.

How well educated must the caregiving nurse be? Practicing nurses feel pressure to know more after they have been pushed into the labor market with brief preparation. It is demands for clinical knowledge from practicing nurses that drive our erratically assembled, remedial, post-basic education efforts, such as BSN completion programs, mandatory continuing education, and tuition support through job benefits.

NURSING KNOWLEDGE

We know that nursing knowledge is made up of six unequal parts: (1) general knowledge about the world and its culture, (2) functional knowledge of social and physical sciences, (3) detailed knowledge of illness, (4) expertise in human behavior in illness and health, (5) expertise in nursing and medical therapeutics, and (6) expert knowledge and teaching capability regarding prevailing standards of health. Because nursing is a practice profession, substantial portions of clinical nursing knowledge are conveyed through protracted expert-to-novice teaching of finely developed skills and understandings. This interactive learning is brilliantly described by Benner et al.[3]

In the last 40 years, our system of conveying nursing knowledge has become fractionalized. Today, faculty who prepare nurses in associate degree programs rarely meet faculty in baccalaureate and masters programs, and faculty who teach doctoral students or midwives or nurse practitioners may never talk to anyone but themselves. Thus the educators of caregiving nurses, future faculty, and researchers do not deliberate together, and there is little involvement of clinical practitioners in educational decisions. How did this happen?

HISTORICAL OVERVIEW

In the 19th century, when nursing came out of the home and into the hospital, nursing care for patients naturally enough imitated domestic or "family" patterns. The nursing superintendent and her assistants held all authority over the nurses, who were mostly pupils in the hospital-owned school. Pupils were organized into a hierarchy, with the oldest directing the youngest. The care of hospital patients was done by inexperienced, tightly supervised, loyal, and interdependent student workers, who came and went with metronome-like regularity.[4]

Private duty in homes and hospitals remained the dominant mode of graduate nursing practice until the late 1930s. Private nurses used skills learned in training, supplemented by journal reading and new information garnered at alumnae meetings or from physicians.[5] Only nurses in public health had access to organized post-basic education in their clinical field. The few other post-basic nursing education programs—the most notable of which was at Teacher's College, Columbia University—prepared nurses for teaching or administration.

THE FAMILY METHOD COLLAPSES

After World War II student nurses were gradually withdrawn from their formerly central role of hospital caregivers, leaving the nurse superintendent to contend with graduate nurses as staff. The authoritarian "family" method of hospital nursing care collapsed. The introduction of graduate nurses caused a major psychologic shift in the system. Although some degree of their learned submissiveness remained, they resented and ultimately refused to accept the child role of the old student-oriented nursing system, in which the head nurse and the supervisor dictated all activity.

A new nursing care system was needed to replace the hierarchical superintendent model, and one was created: "team nursing."[6] Team nursing decentralized leadership but retained the bureaucratic model, extending the service of the professional nurse by making her a manager of others with lesser training and skills: Nurse aides, practical nurses, orderlies, and students. The nursing team leader did not usually select or reward her team members. Nor, except for students, were team members expected to advance to leader status. Nevertheless, the team nursing concept served as a bridge between highly centralized, function-oriented, student-staffed care systems and later, more patient-oriented "primary" care systems staffed by graduate nurses.

A NEW SYSTEM—A NEED FOR MORE KNOWLEDGE

Pressure to improve the quality of nursing care to hospital patients escalated in the late 1950s and 1960s. The care needs of growing numbers of seriously ill, physiologically unstable patients overwhelmed the nurse-conserving team nursing strategy. Nurses, physicians, and hospital administrators turned to a variation on the old private duty nursing concept and gave it a new name—"intensive care." Generally drawn from the best younger nurses, intensive care nurses of the 1960s cared for patients clustered together on the basis of physiologic instability, rather than traditional selectors such as diagnosis, admitting physician, ability to pay, or sex.[7]

Grouping together the most seriously ill patients and naming a select nursing staff to care for them cast the knowledge deficits of the nursing staff in sharp relief. Keenly feeling their lack of essential knowledge, intensive care nurses quickly banded together with their medical colleagues to learn more biomedical science, interpersonal skills, and physical assessment skills. In a few years, on-the-job, ad hoc self-instruction metamorphosed into educational programs sponsored by the federal government's Regional Medical Programs, medical professional groups, and, by the 1970s, the American Association of Critical-Care Nurses. It would be at least a decade, however, before critical care content began to be standard in basic and advanced nursing education programs.

The Education Boom

Intensive or critical care nursing is only one example of the explosive change that occurred in nursing practice in the years between 1960 and 1990. Nurse midwives staked out and occupied their clinical field with the help of satisfied consumers. Nurse practitioners included assessment and clinical management of common health problems in their practice. Psychiatric nurse specialists, spawned by the post-World War II education boom, demonstrated the clinical effectiveness of skilled nursing in care of the mentally ill.

It was in the practice of staff nurses in hospitals and home care that the most fundamental changes occurred. Expectations of staff nurses came to include management of life-support systems, titration of lethal drugs, active participation in selecting therapies, advocacy for patients and families, complex rehabilitation, patient and family education, and multilayered interdisciplinary cooperation.

When team nursing was introduced in the late 1940s and early 1950s, the vast majority of nurses were educated in hospital schools. But demands for better nursing in hospitals and changes in American education were to turn nursing education on its head over the next decades.

After World War II Americans began to insist on broader access to post-high school education. Originally supported by veteran's educational benefits, popular demand was soon reinforced by corporations' needs for new workers in an expanding postwar economy.[8] Later, fear of competition from the Soviet Union after Sputnik (1957) kept up the pressure. Political consensus to commit dollars to education opened colleges and universities to the middle class; it also practically created a new educational phenomenon, the community college.

Placing nursing education programs in community colleges as a way to relocate nursing education out of hospital schools fit this broad reform. Fueled by local pride, a growing tax base, philanthropic support, and public consensus, the community colleges grew and spread; many found nursing programs essential to filling their role as local educational centers.

Meanwhile, the rise of insurance for hospital care and educational subsidies for higher education in nursing conspired to erode hospital training schools. The essential rationale for hospital-based nursing education had been inexpensive, accessible nursing service from students. Widespread hospital insurance made it possible for newly affluent hospitals to pay cash for nursing service rather than ask students to barter their work for education.

And, in reaction to the abysmal treatment of the mentally ill and the lack of professional providers in psychiatry, the National Mental Health Act was passed in 1946. This Act, which supported advanced specialty education for the first time, gave nurses interested in mental health a leg up at all collegiate levels. Other women found the doors to college opened to them through veteran's benefits and state educational subsidies. Armed with these resources, the more career-minded nursing students chose college over hospital-training programs.

Before World War II there were a handful of baccalaureate programs; by 1945 there were 26.[9] After the war both generic programs and postgraduate BS programs grew in number. "Following the money" that became available for nursing education, the greatest increase occurred after 1956, when the first Professional Nurse Traineeship Program under Title Two of the Health Amendment Act provided funds to pursue advanced preparation. The nurses who took advantage of this preparation became the faculties of new programs. In 1956 there were 167 baccalaureate programs nationwide; in 1990 there were nearly 500 baccalaureate programs in the nation's colleges and universities recognized by the National League for Nursing.

The first postwar generation of faculty and deans produced a crucial initial cohort of nurses with higher degrees. However, they were constrained by a diversion of dollars by federal and private funders who felt obliged to salve the political fury of hospitals resisting incursions on their nursing education turf. The first USPHS capitation grants, for instance, helped stave off closure of hospital schools and actually increased their enrollment for a time. Higher degree programs for nurses also received a cool reception from university and college administrators; they were "narrow" professional schools, they brought more women on campus, and they were undeniably expensive.

But the 1960s USPHS Division of Nursing capitation and traineeship grants to nursing provided crucial funding and leverage for fledgling undergraduate women's programs in the nation's male-dominated higher education system. The trickle of nurses graduating with baccalaureate or higher degrees increased to a thin stream. Gradually, the baccalaureate in nursing came to mean generic, clinically focused education, rather than preparation for teaching or administration. Led by the New York State Nurses' Association 1965 resolution, optimistic nurse leaders began a vigorous campaign to claim the baccalaureate degree as the new entry point for professional practice.

Meanwhile, community college nursing programs (ADN), begun in 1952, grew more rapidly than college and university programs. Extraordinary growth of ADN programs caused the associate degree proportion of total registered nurses to nearly triple in the 1970s.[10] In contrast to their cool reception at universities, nursing programs were welcomed by community college presidents and faculty, who saw them as prestigious additions to other offerings.

Proposed as a postwar route to social mobility for the middle and lower classes, community colleges also alleviated pressure on higher degree institutions to allow direct, early access for all qualified applicants to the nation's colleges and universities. Nursing education was unavoidably caught up in the conflicting roles of the community college. Were the new schools avenues to higher education through local, easy access to the liberal arts and sciences? Or were they vocational schools offering terminal degrees and access to skilled labor jobs?[11] Efforts to create transfer programs to ease movement between community and higher degree nursing education institutions were couched in language such as "open curriculum" and "educational ladder" and attracted support and funding during the 1970s. The trend since 1980, however, has been toward greater isolation of associate degree nursing educators from faculty in colleges and universities.

Often more progressive than their hospital school colleagues, associate degree educators insisted that nursing comprised a unified body of knowledge and skills. Education for nursing, they argued, should reflect that knowledge and distinguish semiprofessional and professional levels of practice, rather than simply rotate students through a series of clinical experiences.[12] Nursing faculty in associate degree programs tried hard to articulate levels of nursing knowledge and specify the objectives their graduates would achieve. But distinctions between nurses prepared at the associate degree and baccalaureate levels remained hypothetical until distinctions among nurses in the practice world began to be clarified by critical care nurses, nurse practitioners, midwives, psychiatric nurse clinicians, and other expert nurses.

For 40 years nursing education has been racing to respond to the nation's seemingly insatiable demand for nurses, to catch up with nurses' changing scope of practice, to find faculty and dollars to train beginners and specialists thoroughly and efficiently, and to meet university standards of research and scholarship. All these adaptations were demanded in the midst of a sweeping relocation of the education enterprise—out of hospital-based schools and into community colleges and universities. Tuning the education of nurses to the realities and potentials of late 20th century nursing practice absorbed the energies of two generations of clinicians and educators.

THE CONTEMPORARY SCENE

We think that knowing this history helps clarify the interlocking, reciprocal, enhancing, delaying, and diverting effects of clinical, institutional, and societal change on nursing education and practice. Moreover, the remarkable changes wrought during the last 40 years should give us a strong sense of confidence and direction.

Nevertheless, unlike any other profession or educated occupational group, and despite recommendations from every report written about nursing, we are fast approaching the 21st century without an agreement on educational entry to our profession. We can no longer delay dealing with the questions surrounding preparation of the staff nurse caregiver. It is time to reexamine the numbers of students in each type of program preparing for the RN license and look at the implications of recruitment for those programs. We need to match student ability with the type of program offered. We need to attend to the widely recognized annual imbalance between the number of graduates from associate degree programs and baccalaureate programs.

DOCTORAL EDUCATION FOR ENTRY

Some nursing leaders dealt with the problem by proposing doctoral education for entry into the profession. The group who held this view was small but bright, articulate, and influential. In the light of slow progress in attaining the baccalaureate as entry level, proposals for the doctorate seem to obscure the real problems of the profession and the patients it serves.

From the first decades of the 20th century, nurses and others have studied and made recommendations for change, upgrading, differentiation, and clarity. Most of these studies and recommendations held certain commonalities. First, they assumed the baccalaureate was the preferred degree for entry into the profession, and, second (and most important), they have considered the *occupation* (i.e., the work of nurses) as well as the *profession* of nursing. If one examines only the profession of nursing, there is little argument with those who advocate the doctorate for entry. Indeed, the knowledge and maturity requirements of a complex discipline, the status conferred and implied by the doctoral degree, and the parity issue with medicine are compelling arguments for a truly differentiating credential between the "professional" nurse and all others who are involved in the nursing arena. But there's the rub: Nursing is an *occupation* that promises to care for people in knowledgeable, compassionate, and direct ways.

Implicit in the idea of graduate education for entry into the profession is a declaration that associate degree or diploma preparation is enough for most first-line nurse caregivers. The notion that the doctorally prepared nurse will be our basic professional caregiver refutes economics, the work and lifestyle choices of such people, and history's lessons. Let us remember that demands for nurses confounded previous efforts to differentiate between baccalaureate, associate degree, and diploma nurses. Demand for nurses created many of the problems we are now trying to solve. We believe nursing should be cautious before embracing elitist solutions that might sound the death knell for a professional base and the self-image of the practicing staff nurse.

BACCALAUREATE EDUCATION FOR ENTRY

The argument for making the BSN the norm for personal caregiving rests on the nation's need for (1) broadly capable generalist caregivers to practice in a variety of settings; (2) a pool from which people may be drawn who are capable of advanced training as specialists, leaders, researchers; (3) productive collaborators holding educational preparation similar to other health care workers; and (4) an approach that builds on prevailing patterns of elementary, junior high, and high school curriculums. Most important, asserting the baccalaureate as the norm for nursing practice recognizes the reality of nursing as an occupation (i.e., a vital work serving the public), as well as a profession (i.e., a living body of knowledge and skills).

To ensure safe patient care, at the least, the proportion of nurses prepared at the baccalaureate level must exceed those prepared at lower levels. Shortages are increasing in faculty positions. New data indicate reductions in student numbers at the masters' level. Clearly, the nation's pool of bedside caregivers requires an infusion of BSN-prepared nurses who can care for the complex, physiologically/ psychologically unstable people crowding our hospitals and seeking professional care in their homes. Nurses need in-depth science and arts education, excellent clinical experience, and the time to absorb both. Professional education provides needed breadth and flexibility for students preparing for a lifetime career and inculcates the habit of life-long-learning—a crucial part of nursing culture.

The baccalaureate degree in nursing is legitimate and coherent. It meets the obligation of the profession to produce safe, competent, and productive workers and permits the profession to reproduce itself normally, that is, through university graduate programs. Imagine a scenario with no direct route to nursing through the normal American educational system. The gap among those who profess to be nurses would exceed that extant between nurses and physicians and other health professionals, would discourage applicants who view nursing as a practice discipline, would sharply decrease the pool of nurses prepared to enter clinical specialist graduate programs, and would have disastrous effects on future faculty preparation.

In short, the impact of undermining the baccalaureate from both higher and lower levels would be to separate the practice of nursing from its theoretical proponents. The ideology of nursing would be beautiful, perhaps, but it would be divorced from the reality of the workplace.

The entry of high school graduates, of any age, into the system of higher education is the standard for engineers, accountants, business people, lawyers, physicians, and others; it is becoming the standard for nursing. But the proportions of nurses we are preparing at the baccalaureate level belie this commonality. The numbers of students in associate degree programs continue to exceed those entering baccalaureate programs.

In its "1990 Report to the President and Congress," the Department of Health and Human Services forecast that by the year 2000 there will be half as many BSN and higher degree nurses and nearly twice as many associate degree nurses as needed. These projections worsen over time for baccalaureate and higher degree nurses. For the year 2000 they show a deficiency of nearly 700,000 prepared at the baccalaureate and higher degree level and an excess of nearly 200,000 prepared at the associate degree level (Figures 1 and 2).[13]

In 1994–95, 31,254 basic students were graduated from baccalaureate nursing programs, and almost double that number (58,749) were graduated from associate degree programs. Even more serious, enrollments in 1996 were 103,213 basic students in BSN programs, 122,242 in ADN programs, and 12,789 in diploma programs. Recognizing that ADN students graduate in 2 to 3 years, an almost 20% difference in enrollment must be approximately doubled to see the eventual mismatch between preparation and need.[2]

In recent years, demand for baccalaureate prepared nurses from hospital nursing employers has put associate degree graduates in a catch-up situation educationally, making them dependent on the innovativeness and receptiveness of baccalaureate programs. The resulting unplanned articulation of poorly matched nurse education programs tends to be inefficient, expensive, and a source of irritation for students and faculty alike. Many associate degree graduates are turned off, get a poor deal, choose the wrong degree completion programs, then, from a clinical practice viewpoint, find themselves with a not-very-useful baccalaureate degree.

Education and experience do materially influence what and how much nurses know, and that makes a difference to the health and well-being of nurses' patients. The vast majority of able students with the resources to do so should choose, or be guided to, the baccalaureate after high school.* A more coherent, better under-

---

*We are not discussing either direct entry master's degree programs for nonnurse college graduates or fast track BSN/MSN for the same population. We endorse these programs, given quality clinical and theoretical preparation. Further, we do not discuss degree completion programs for RNs.

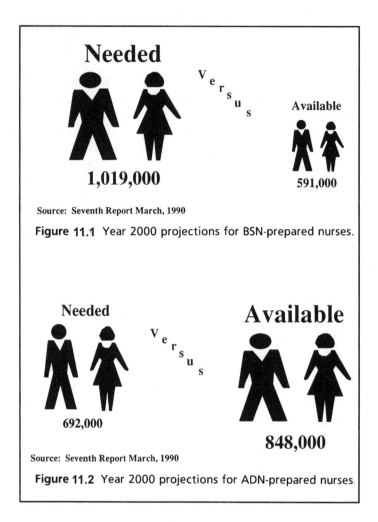

Source: Seventh Report March, 1990

Figure 11.1 Year 2000 projections for BSN-prepared nurses.

Source: Seventh Report March, 1990

Figure 11.2 Year 2000 projections for ADN-prepared nurses.

FIGURES 11.1 & 11.2

stood, fairer educational system can be devised. Designing such a system will require candid talk between ADN and BSN/MSN faculty.

As others have noted before, it is crucial that we distinguish our social equity arguments from our obligation to prepare quality practitioners at each level.[14] Associate degree education has been a vital point of entry for older students, some minorities, and nontraditional students. But there are classist, racist, and gender implications inherent in that position. With appropriate guidance and financial aid, future nurses would achieve true social mobility via baccalaureate education.

A NEW SYSTEM

We propose a plan that recognizes our already existing population in nursing without prejudice, appreciates past attempts to solve these dilemmas, assumes membership of the largest group we are now preparing—the associate degree graduate—in the nursing body politic, and provides a cadre of professionals without the impossible task of disenfranchisement.

DIRECT TRANSFER LINKAGE PROGRAM

First, we must expand access to generic baccalaureate programs and find strategies to strengthen them financially and educationally. There are at least four essential aspects to this task, some of which are underway: (1) agreement on theoretical and clinical content with the support of the American Association of Colleges of Nursing (AACN) and the National League for Nursing (NLN); (2) grant support for consultation services from AACN and NLN for programs to meet accepted standards; (3) support for faculty sharing in appropriate areas; and (4) financial support for students from state and federal governments, foundations, and employers.

Second, we must find ways to improve the linkages between community colleges and baccalaureate programs in nursing and build strong nurse associate programs. At least three options are needed. All will require funded demonstration and evaluation; institutions testing the new options will cease offering the ADN program.

A prime target for change is to increase community college and senior college programs that encourage direct transfer of liberal arts and science courses from community colleges to BSN programs. This is a neglected but unarguable option that should present little difficulty in implementation. It requires collaboration of senior college(s) and community college(s) faculty and assumes that completion of the requirements for professional nursing and licensure occurs only at the baccalaureate level.

The direct transfer linkage program includes a selected group of prenursing liberal arts and sciences courses agreed on jointly by one or more senior colleges in collaboration with community college faculty. Transfer of the students into senior college is guaranteed, on satisfactory completion of the prenursing program. Financial aid designated for nursing students would commence once the student is in the nursing component.

PARTNERSHIP PROJECT

The second program is a partnership experiment and also consists of a transferable program of study. The new program would be housed in a partnership between one or more junior colleges, and one or more senior colleges, with consultation from nursing administrators and state planning bodies. Student transfer between partner colleges would be permitted after either the first or the second year. The first 2 years at the community college would be planned together and all first-year courses would be identical. These courses would be offered at a level that would permit full transferability. The second year would include basic educational courses and focus, in nursing, on one clinical option, planned together, and totally transferrable to the senior college or a consortium of senior colleges. After the 2 years, the graduate would be permitted to test in the clinical option and obtain a position as a nursing technician. Choices might eventually include gerontologic care, maternal health, child health, or psychiatric nursing. Only two would be permitted during the trial period. Thus the student in the transferable program of study would, at the end of 2 years, have a means of self-support as a health care worker and access to a planned program leading to the BSN.

NURSE ASSOCIATE PROGRAM

A third and crucial option will be a terminal program, with a base in arts and science and introductory nursing courses in the first year and a focus on theory and clinical work in long-term care, specifically in nursing homes, in the second. Community college nursing faculty are already making great strides in this vital area of care; the location of new programs would depend on the availability of faculty in gerontologic nursing offering their talents to meet this purpose.* Associate nurses prepared in these programs would help resolve problems of quality among assistive nursing personnel in the nation's nursing homes. Many states are already mandating education for assistive personnel in nursing homes. For this program to be implemented current resources should be committed to the nurse associate program and approval from necessary government and voluntary bodies must be obtained.

Because of the necessity to move large systems, these options must be mounted as trials with support from one or more major foundations. Basic to all options is the requirement that regional advisement programs be established and that financial aid programs be practical enough to enable those students who are eligible to enter baccalaureate programs directly, or after 1 or 2 years of pre-nursing education.

Essential to these initiatives is increased productivity from our BSN programs through expanded access and strategies to strengthen them academically and financially. Increased productivity will require schools to recruit a diverse body of students through financial and programmatic incentives, provision of consultation services to schools to improve curriculum offerings, support for regional faculty sharing, and higher levels of financial aid for students.

SUMMARY AND RECOMMENDATIONS

We propose to end the bifurcation of professional nursing. Our strategies for the 21st century include several new programs that have potential to meet the needs for an associate nurse, solve the political problems of the community college for students and money, offer employers a less confused and potentially less expensive caregiving staff, and provide a viable career for many men and women. At the same time, we can address the vital goal of increasing our output of baccalaureate-prepared nurses.

---

*The W. K. Kellogg Foundation—sponsored Community College/Nursing Home Partnership and the Robert Wood Johnson Foundation Teaching Nursing Home Project showed conclusively that faculty and long-term care facilities can forge creative, productive alliances to improve care and educate caregivers.

TABLE 11.1   ACCESS TO THE BACCALAUREATE

DIRECT TRANSFER LINKAGE PROGRAM

Direct transfer of liberal arts and sciences only

   a. guided program of prenursing arts and sciences selected jointly by one or more senior colleges in collaboration with community college faculty
   b. assumption of transfer into senior college on satisfactory completion of prenursing program
   c. financial aid for students once in nursing component

PARTNERSHIP PROJECT

A regional transfer program-partnership between one or more community colleges and one or more senior colleges.

   a. all first-year courses identical: transfer possible to senior college if desired
   b. second year: continue liberal arts and sciences and include one clinical option, transferable to senior college. This could include gerontologic care, maternal health, child health, or psychiatric nursing
   c. choice of option determines which prerequisites must be offered
   d. only two clinical options permitted during the trial
   e. student may test in clinical option to become employable "nursing technician" in _____ nursing.
   f. access to senior college guaranteed on successful completion of course work.

NURSE ASSOCIATE PROGRAM

   a. base in arts and sciences and nursing skills
   b. focus in second year on long-term care (nursing homes)
   c. consultation and faculty sharing, especially in gerontology
   d. RN program closed; resources committed to nurse associates
   e. approval from necessary government and voluntary bodies

We recommend that trials be mounted in at least five states. A 6-year period of experimentation and demonstration will be necessary to permit completion of four classes and evaluation of the various options. The trials would require cooperation from the state boards of nursing, from the Joint Commission on Accreditation of Health Care Organizations, from regulatory agencies, and from the legislatures of the five states so that some form of license or work permit would be guaranteed to participants testing satisfactorily in the 2-year clinical option.

Results of these trials will provide information and experience to support or refute the eventual closing of RN associate degree programs and, at the same time, have the potential of providing skilled associate nurses who can meet many specific needs. The transfer programs would permit nursing to continue to be a field that opens its doors to all segments of society and permit upward mobility in a sound way, protective of both students and the public. The terminal program offers new workers an effective, fair opportunity to get into the health field and safeguards the public from untrained caregivers. The question of honesty in education is a real one; we must provide the public with a worker prepared for an increasingly complex world with more than a smattering of nursing knowledge. And nursing must accept its responsibility to prepare associate workers.

These demonstrations or experiments would provide answers to three questions that have nagged at nursing and health care for decades: What are the most functional relationships between professional nurses and assistive personnel? (We tried to look at this question when the licensed practical nurse appeared after World War II, but nursing leaders did not support the LPN and the question faded away to legalisms.) What are the capacities and linkages that work best between community colleges and universities in preparing nurses? (Experiments in the 1970s tested some of the possibilities but need to be recalled and reexamined.) How can we articulate and realize our goal of high-quality nursing professionals at the same time we retain and fulfill our goal of access to nursing for all?

The public assumes we will meet and solve our dilemma. Notwithstanding the difficulties we face in making our educational system more coherent and productive, we are optimistic that we can do so. After all, we have already created a public and private enterprise that can produce more than 70,000 nurses a year; we now have an academic superstructure with a good chance of survival in the nations' universities and colleges; we have a large press; and, most important, we have a restless, energizing demand for our product—the American nurse.

ENDNOTES

1. Hart, P. D. (1989). A nationwide survey of attitudes toward health care and nursing. Washington: Peter D. Hart Associates.
1a. Findings from National Sample Survey of Registered Nurses, DHHS, Rockville, MD, March 1996.

2. Nursing Data Review. New York: National League for Nursing unpublished telephone interview, approximate data, March 2000.
3. Benner, P. (1984). From novice to expert—excellence and power in clinical nursing practice. Menlo Park, California: Addison-Wesley.
4. Lynaugh, J., & Fagin, C. (1988). Nursing comes of age. *Image, 20,* 184–190.
5. Reverby, S. (1983). Something besides waiting: The politics of private duty nursing reform in the Depression. In E. Lagemann (Ed.), *Nursing history new perspectives, new possibilities.* New York: Teacher's College Press.
6. Lambertsen, E. (1953). *Nursing team organization and functioning.* New York: Teachers College.
7. Fairman, J. We need more nurses: The development of intensive care units and the nursing shortage, 1955–1965. Presented to the Annual Conference, American Association for the History of Nursing, Galveston, Texas, Sept. 28, 1990.
8. U.S. President's Commission on Higher Education. (1948). Higher education for American democracy. New York: Harper Brothers. [First released in 1947 and commonly called the Truman Commission.]
9. National League for Nursing Education. (1945). Courses in clinical nursing for graduate nurses, basic assumptions and guiding principles-basic courses-advanced courses. Pamphlet # 1. New York: National League for Nursing Education.
10. Schoen, D., & Schoen, R. (1985). A life table analysis of the labor force participation of U.S. nurses, 1949–1980. *Research in Nursing and Health, 8,* 105–116.
11. Brint, S., & Karabel, J. *The diverted dream—community colleges and the promise of educational opportunity in America, 1900–1985.* New York: Oxford University Press.
12. Montag, M., & Gotkin, L. (1966). Community college education for nursing. In B. Bullough & V. Bullough (Eds.), *Issues in nursing.* New York: Springer Publishing.
13. U.S. Public Health Service. Nursing—Seventh Report to the President and Congress on the Status of Health Personnel (1990). Washington: USPHS.
14. Waters, V. (1975). Curriculum problems in the open curriculum. In C. Lenburg, *Open learning and career mobility in nursing.* St. Louis: CV Mosby.

Based on a keynote presentation at the University of Michigan School of Nursing's Centennial Celebration in May 1991.

Historical research for this essay was supported, in part, by grants (J.E.L.) from the W. K. Kellogg Foundation and the American Association of Critical-Care Nurses. This essay represents the views of the authors only. It does not report the position of any professional organization.

CHAPTER TWELVE

Institutionalizing Faculty Practice

Claire M. Fagin

The nursing profession since its inception has been preoccupied with links between nursing education and nursing practice. More recently, efforts to institutionalize faculty practice have received considerable attention, focusing particularly on three institutions: Case Western Reserve University, Rush-Presbyterian, and the University of Rochester. Despite this attention, there has been little replication or emulation of these examples of unification or clinical models. This chapter will attempt to explain this by placing efforts to institutionalize practice in the context of their historical antecedents. It will also describe developments at the University of Pennsylvania in what we are calling a partnership.

HISTORICAL ANTECEDENTS

The pre-education period of nursing training did not offer examples of faculty practice by any definition because they offered few exam-

Note: This was published in *Nursing Outlook*, Vol. 34, No. 3, May/June 1986. It is reprinted here with permission.

ples of *faculty*. Teaching and teachers barely existed, and the focus was, for the most part, on devoted, self-sacrificing service. Clearly, historical perspectives on this subject do not begin with organized nursing service or training school development.

On the other hand, current developments have been influenced by beliefs from educational institutions. In 1932, the National League of Nursing Education, through its newly developed department of studies, published a landmark report, *An Activity Analysis of Nursing*.[1] Focusing on efficiency, it described the practice of nursing as a series of activities and became the "basis for . . . curriculum development" throughout the country. Similar studies followed. These researchers (notably Isabel Stewart at Teachers College) were intrigued with the work of Lillian and Frank Gilbreth, the American efficiency engineers whose management methods became synonymous with productivity. Stewart and her colleagues believed that their approach, focusing on scientific organization and structure, would regularize nursing and ensure safety, efficiency, and the legitimacy of nursing's presence in hospitals.[2] This perspective gave birth to many nursing movements, penultimately to team nursing and possibly to our current view of unification.

Meanwhile, Virginia Henderson was trying to make a case that the way for nursing to legitimize itself was not through scientific management methods but rather by asking questions about clinical practice. So she set out to examine the problems of the day and nursing's best approach to their resolution. This dichotomy of approach—that is, the conflict between viewing structure as the means to accomplish our goals versus focusing on the best and most compelling ideas about nursing care—is still at the root of some of our dilemmas in institutionalizing practice. The revolutionary step taken by Dorothy Smith at the University of Florida represents the first move to close the educational/practice gap and her belief that structure was the way to do it.

In 1956 Dorothy Smith was recruited to be dean of the College of Nursing for the University of Florida's new academic health center. She accepted the position after the administration agreed that she would also be the director of nursing service. The patterns of organization at both Rush and Rochester can be seen as based on the University of Florida example. Smith's goals were: To introduce an intellectual and clinical nursing role that would influence people about the nature of nursing; to guarantee faculty practice; to develop nursing systems and a data base; to develop an educational hierarchy in nursing service and to obtain power. She "developed the structure for power and had the power when the institution was small enough to be cohesive."[3] By 1972 Smith had lost power, and she resigned that year, at age 59, to the great loss of the nursing profession. In this case, structure provided neither power nor safety. Despite wide admiration for her accomplishments, she was left at the mercy of changed professional relationships and environmental conditions that increased vulnerability for her and her structure. However, Smith left an indelible impression on all who knew her, and she endowed the University of Florida students of her era with a sense of the power, significance, and beauty of the nursing profession.

CONTINUATION AND HEIGHTENING OF INTEREST

While Dorothy Smith was aiming to institute an intellectual role for nurses at the University of Florida that would focus on problem solving and would exemplify and build nursing knowledge, Rozella Schlotfeldt was planning an organization that would be built on academic leadership of nursing. The faculty of Case Western Reserve University approved this plan in 1961, just three years after the University of Florida opened its hospital. The academic leadership design, quite different from unification, was in its planning and development stages while Smith was beginning her innovations. Many current schemes for faculty/clinician appointments seem to have been influenced by the Case Western Reserve example. Termed "academic leadership" for nursing, it allows faculty the right to nominate candidates for "agreed upon leadership positions in . . . relevant service agencies."[4] Following the Florida and Case Western Reserve experiences were the innovations of Luther Christman at Rush-Presbyterian University and Loretta Ford at the University of Rochester. Both have been well described in the literature, but from the standpoint of replication several points should be noted. Rush-Presbyterian University is a free-standing medical center. The College of Nursing, in its effort to accomplish multiple goals, has its own distinct policies for appointments and retention of faculty, which do not include provisions for tenure. Nursing faculties in more traditional universities are not likely to accept this stance. Thus, while Rush's clinical model may be successful in its own distinct setting, it would not seem to be an appropriate model for most universities.

At the University of Rochester, a new organizational structure labeled "a unification model" was established in 1972, " . . . with nursing assuming authority and accountability in the three areas of nursing education, practice, and research."[5] While this structure has had many successes in making organizational changes, problems in meeting its multiple goals have been well described.[6]

These institutions have provided the rest of us with extraordinary stimulation. They have moved the profession forward by raising the visibility of professional nursing practice, giving legitimacy to faculty practice, demonstrating the possibilities of autonomy for nurses and collaborative practice with physicians and others, and winning the support of powerful advocates on the national scene. They took on the profession at the height of the education/practice gap and have provided the impetus for the development of a wide variety of faculty practice endeavors. But in spite of the enormous professional gains stimulated by these institutions, the implicit or explicit enshrining of their organizational design has often stood in the way of the development of different patterns that might be as effective in institutionalizing faculty practice and more widely replicable.

Considerable progress has been made in closing the gap between education and practice. But from the standpoint of institutionalizing practice, unless this progress addresses the multiple missions of our universities and clinical agencies, there will be no models or prototypes. There are currently many examples of faculty practice in community settings such as nursing centers, midwifery/birthing centers, and primary care practices. The majority of university programs have some faculty in shared positions with hospitals and other agencies. The percentage of time spent in the various roles (usually teaching and practice) varies as does the method of cost sharing and the style of employment. In general, however, these shared appointments are teaching/practice roles. There are a few faculty practice examples that encourage both clinical leadership on the part of faculty and research on nursing phenomena. These examples, which recognize the essential role of research in faculty practice, are an important development in nursing's maturity. The Robert Wood Johnson Teaching-Nursing Home and Clinical Scholar programs may be the paradigms for the future of faculty practice, much as the RWJF Nurse Faculty Program in Primary Care served among the initial stimuli.

It is interesting to contrast nursing's concern for faculty practice with medicine's. The education/practice gap is frequently traced to nursing's choice not to follow the lead of medical education when it moved from its apprentice training system but instead to follow the teacher's college methodology of clinical practice as laboratory.

Yet if we examine the medical model as our starting place, it becomes evident that our signals somehow became crossed or our priorities skewed. The theoretical basis for change in medical education was adoption of a research approach instead of a practice approach. Their move from the past was characterized by a view of the medical school as " . . . a place where medicine is not only taught but studied."[7] Our initial view of *nursing school* was a place where nursing should be taught and learned. Our more current trend is to see nursing school as a place where nursing is both taught and *practiced.* This underlying theme may be a more crucial problem than we have recognized and may be one explanation of why we have not yet developed explicitly replicable models.

THE PENN EXPERIENCE

The process and progress in institutionalizing practice at the University of Pennsylvania has been characterized by all the problems and pitfalls I have described. Our perspective has been affected by nursing's history, the notion that we could emulate existing models, and the belief in structure. We have been struggling with the idea of institutionalizing faculty practice or merging the complementary missions of the School of Nursing and the Division of Nursing at the Hospital of the University of Pennsylvania since 1977, when the first committee was formed to develop a "model." The process was propelled forward by the appointment of a new director of nursing (associate administrator for nursing) as associate dean of the School of Nursing in 1982.

The School of Nursing's stated mission is to be at the cutting edge of the discipline of nursing by developing and strengthening the knowledge base for nursing practice through research, by providing excellence in the quality of the school's baccalaureate and graduate programs, and by developing leaders in the disciplines among its faculty and graduates. The Division of Nursing at the Hospital of the University of Pennsylvania aims to be at the forefront of many advances in clinical nursing and its practice mission requires that it encourage and sustain theory and practice pertinent to the nursing care needs of patients with complex medical problems. The faculty of the School of Nursing therefore focus on the generation and dissemination of nursing knowledge, while the clinicians of the Division of Nursing focus on the use of nursing knowledge.[8]

Several conclusions emerged from this lengthy study.

- It was determined that a partnership, in addressing the complementary missions of nursing at the university, would provide teaching and research environments where nursing theory and clinical practice would enrich each other for the mutual benefit of students, patients, faculty, and staff.
- An important aspect of the university's structure is that the dean is relatively autonomous. It was deemed unwise to give the dean responsibility for the operation of nursing care at the hospital, thereby making the nursing dean responsible to persons in equal or lower positions.
- Nursing research was considered of prime importance to the partnership. While this should be true in every university model of unification, it is particularly true at Penn because of the emphasis on research throughout the university. A leadership school in any discipline cannot exist at such a university unless it reflects common values. While faculty at Penn are engaged in a wide variety of research, including philosophy, ethics, and history, the majority are engaged in clinical research and thus involved in activities that are exemplary of faculty practice.

Because of the highly academic nature of our institution, the committee recognized that the partnership must begin at leadership levels and focus on those eligible for faculty appointments. Early partnership documents described elaborate organizational designs for the school and division, with newly named departments (predominantly service driven) and a strong focus on the chairman role, analogous to the medical model and the institutions previously cited.

Draft proposals were widely shared and committees solicited faculty, administration and nursing staff input. Concerns were expressed about budget decisions, hiring and firing of key personnel, relationships with key administrators, and implications of the partnership for the entire nursing staff, not only the leaders. The faculty questioned possible diminution of their autonomy, an overemphasis on clinical research as the only research of merit, and the assumption of governance by new bodies that might interfere with the current system of faculty governance.

During the lengthy planning phase, many shared activities had accelerated. Faculty practice opportunities in such areas as research, primary care, gerontological care, midwifery, and critical care had already been implemented and plans were made to bring the Center for Nursing Research of the School of Nursing and the Inquiry and Development program of the Hospital of the University of Pennsylvania closer together. Further, collaborative arrangements in staff development have been instituted and faculty practice arrangements with other major clinical sites have been formalized. All of these activities were *independent* of structural changes.

In revising the plan, most of us came to believe we had leaned too heavily on merger and unification and focused too little on partnership while using all three words. The three principal goals— clinical excellence, developing a research and scholarly base, and provision of excellent educational programs—may be interrelated, but the divergences are greater than the common ground. Our focus on merger or unification seems to have been influenced more by a fourth, less stated goal than by the three major goals pertaining to the clinical and academic setting. This goal is empowerment of practicing nurses and the nursing profession, a legitimate although somewhat paradoxical aim given our current realities. On one hand, faculty—though themselves not familiar with the practice setting— state expectations of students that include leadership, autonomy, and change in the patient care arena. Their expectations also include risk taking, which the faculty themselves have never successfully experienced. On the other hand, in the practice arenas, nurses are employees in bureaucratic organizations and often see themselves as relatively powerless to take the risks that accomplish change because of the perceived insecurity of their jobs.

This fourth major goal, therefore, is to raise the power level of nurses at large, to unify the body politic of the profession, to instill a oneness of professional values, and to expand the leadership group. This goal is directly related to nursing and the nursing professional ideal and indirectly to patients or students. It is also the goal, whether covertly or overtly stated, that arouses the most intense reactions during the development and maintenance of the process of reorganization. It is this fourth goal that provides the major argument for unification of nursing education and nursing practice, because it can be argued on the basis of our own observation and the study of others that the other three goals in complex organizations are more differentiated than not.[9]

Currently, medical schools and hospitals are reexamining their organizational structures and we can expect this trend to continue in the coming years. As stresses related to cost containment increase, the organizational efficiencies of the matrix structure and blurring of task differentiation will be subjected to hard examination. There is recurring pressure on expert medical practitioners to *practice* and bring in revenues that support other functions of the medical school. By the same token, university constraints on faculty permanence and promotion are not easing. Thus the assumption of greater differentiation in the practice/education missions of professional disciplines must at least be explored.

THE CLINICIAN-EDUCATOR FACULTY POSITION

We have come to believe strongly, with others, that organizational designs within the hospital structure(s) are only one aspect of promoting the multiple and often dichotomous missions of the institutions involved. In many instances, *position* design may be more functional than *organization* design. We have also come to believe that a position critical to the achievement of all four goals is something akin to what we call the clinician-educator (C.E.) faculty appointment.

At Penn, full-time, fully credentialed faculty make up the standing faculty. The standing faculty includes faculty with tenure or in tenure probationary status, and clinician-educators. The first type are investigator/educators whose primary interests lie in clinical or basic research. The clinician-educators, whose interests lie in clinical practice, also make a significant contribution to the educational program. Clinician-educators are expected to engage in scholarly activities, including publications, and their teaching is likely to be practice-oriented. This definition implies assigning greater weight to teaching and clinical or practice competence rather than to research when evaluating candidates for appointment and promotion. The principal features of the C.E. appointments are that persons in this category share all rights and privileges of other School of Nursing faculty except voting on tenure and on compensation of tenured faculty; appointees may seek adjudication of unresolved grievances through the established mechanisms of the Grievance Commission and the school's Committee on Academic Freedom and Responsibility as is appropriate to the circumstances. Faculty choosing the C.E. track have 10 years to achieve the rank of associate professor.

It is important to note that teaching, research, and practice *can* occur in both standing faculty positions, but the emphasis on each of these roles is expected to vary from one position to another. The appointment and promotion process acknowledges these differences. It seems to us that such a diverse and well-informed faculty has the greatest potential for developing excellence in its educational program: A faculty in which some members primarily practice, some primarily do research, and both communicate their work in the interest of building their own and their students' knowledge.

PROBLEMS IN IMPLEMENTATION

Negotiations proved most difficult in the area of academic rights and privileges and access to university grievance procedures. While the agency retains the right to discontinue a contract for the service of a clinician-educator, the mechanisms used to do so are subject to review under university policies. These policies may have different rights, privileges, and mechanisms by which recourse can be sought if violations of those rights seem to have occurred.

And yet, if we truly believe that nurses who are excellent practitioners need the same freedoms to explore, to report their findings, and to speak out as do tenure-track standing faculty, then these policies must be a part of any university arrangement for long-term faculty opportunities. It is in this area that the whole appointment structure can make the greatest impact on nursing.

Opposition to such a faculty design may come from several quarters. Some may be concerned that teaching will take on secondary status to both research and practice. However, in most major universities, teaching of a high quality is expected but is never interchangeable with scholarship. Those who believe all faculty should be excellent clinicians will look askance at the investigator-educator. That attitude may serve to impede research efforts among the faculty. While scholarly programs specifically related to patient care do demand that the investigator keep abreast of current care, there are other areas of research and scholarship that do not require the "laying on of hands." Historical and philosophical studies, laboratory studies, the testing of some theories, methodological studies, and many others are not negatively influenced by the fact that the investigator does not practice. Nor is the teaching of these investigators negatively influenced by their lack of current clinical excellence as long as they are given appropriate teaching assignments. Additional questions may be raised if the practice design is seen as quintessentially academic and out of keeping with the hierarchical and bureaucratic organization common in the practice area. However, clinical faculty and clinician-educators, while having the collegiality and protection of an academic environment and its grievance system, will have a contract to perform in a specified clinical role according to specific guidelines and standards of excellence. The clinical practice goal is discrete and measurable in its outcome, and freedom and autonomy are accompanied by accountability. The ingredients of our plan therefore focus on promotion of functioning to meet common and discrete goals through partnership where all leaders are protected by the rules governing academic freedom.

CONCLUSIONS

As we look to the future, any new design for institutionalizing practice must be accompanied by a plan for evaluation of outcomes in the stated goals of the organization—in this case the four primary goals in education, research, nursing practice and professionalism.

Many new patterns of faculty practice as well as the unified patterns of organization have not been studied rigorously. This is a deficit and must be addressed if we are to convert more adherents to any scheme. As we move on to the future we must take a clearer look at missions and goals and determine roles and positions that meet these goals, even if they do not fit into a perfectly designed organizational structure. Overly heavy stress on structure creates the risk that practice mission and goals will subsume other missions; that the university mission and goals will subsume other missions; or that neither mission will be well served. Other possibilities include placing paramount, if covert, emphasis on the professional mission. Empowerment of nurses is a goal to be obtained only, in my opinion, in the context of our major missions of education, research, and practice. A university's primary missions are research and education. Research must result from any endeavor in which faculty are engaged. Faculty practice designs that do not reflect the research agenda are doomed from the start. Descriptions of heroic efforts are inspiring, but not sufficient to maintain themselves after the heroic leaders are gone and certainly not sufficient for replication, especially when one considers the heroism required.

Thus any pattern adopted currently must be flexible enough to fit the vast variety of circumstances and settings in which nursing education and nursing practice occur and must be sufficiently *tested* and *recorded* to be maintained and understood. We believe the key to meeting the goals of institutionalizing faculty practice is the guarantee of academic freedom within the context of a university-wide appointment and governance system. It has potential for uniting people rather than organizations, in behalf of some shared and some discrete goals. It makes them partners in what Giammatti calls "a spirit that transcends the letter of stated principles . . . commitment to free inquiry . . . a spirit of collegiality and . . . a shared sense of respect for the trusteeship of these values."[10] This is what we are striving for in nursing. Given the current and increasing strength of our group, its commitment, the leadership ability of faculty, clinicians, and administrators of educational and practice environments, we can achieve it.

ENDNOTES

1. Lambertson, E. C. (1958). *Education for nursing leadership.* Philadelphia: J. B. Lippincott Co., p. 27.
2. Stewart, I. M. (1919, June). Possibilities of standardization in nursing technique. *Modern Hospital, 12,* 451–454.
3. Smith, D. M. (1964, Feb.). Myth and method in nursing practice. *American Journal of Nursing, 64,* 68–72.
4. Schlotfeldt, R. M. (1981). The development of a model for unifying nursing practice and nursing education. In L. H. Aiken (Ed.), *Health policy and nursing practice* (pp. 218–229). New York: McGraw-Hill Book Co.
5. Ford, L. C. (1981). The University of Rochester model. In T. Keenan and others (Eds.), *Nurses and Doctors, Their Education and Practice* (p. 69). Cambridge, MA: Oelgeschlager, Gunn & Hain Publishers.
6. *Ibid.,* pp. 69–83.
7. Stevens, R. (1971). *American medicine and the public interest* (p. 58). New Haven, CT: Yale University Press.
8. University of Pennsylvania, School of Nursing and the Hospital of the University of Pennsylvania, Division of Nursing. (1984, April). *Partnership in Nursing.* Philadelphia, The University.
9. Charns, M. P., et al. (1977). *Organizing Multiple Function Professionals in Academic Medical Centers* (pp. 71–88). (Reprint No. 753) Pittsburgh, Pa, Graduate School of Industrial Administration, Carnegie Mellon University.
10. Giammatti, B. A. *Free Market and Free Inquiry: The University, Industry, and Cooperative Research.* Paper presented at Partners in the Research Enterprise: A National Conference on University, Corporate Relations in Science and Technology, held at University of Pennsylvania, Philadelphia, Dec. 15, 1982.

PART THREE

Making a Difference—
One Example

Introduction

One of the most exciting aspects of working at Clinical Center, National Institutes of Health during its early development was that it drew visitors from throughout the United States and all over the world. Every Institute was staffed with leaders in all of the health professions who were at the cutting edge of their respective fields in research and clinical interventions. Some of the visitors came to see what was going on, while others came to share their own innovative work with us. One of the latter was James Robertson from Tavistock Clinic in England who was a colleague of psychiatrist John Bowlby and who had just completed a film titled, "A Two Year Old Goes to Hospital."

Robertson showed the film which depicted the experiences of a young child, separated from parents for a brief hospitalization, and it showed her emotions in startlingly vivid terms. The film made a deep impression on me and stimulated much reading about separation in wartime written by Anna Freud, as well as the major work on the subject by Bowlby, "Maternal Care and the Growth of Love." I was also very familiar with the new research on dependency which was taking place at NIH at that time.

My experiences at Children's Hospital in Washington, D.C. provided living examples of what Robertson had shown in the film and later when I was teaching at New York University I used his work and that of Freud and Bowlby in my courses. When our first son Joshua was eighteen months old he was hospitalized for emergency surgery for an inguinal hernia. The first rule we needed to observe was to leave the hospital so the staff could get on with its work. Since I was so imbued with the separation literature and had spread the word to my husband Sam, we were determined that one or the other of us would remain full time with Josh. We took turns and to the dismay of nurses, physicians, and security, each of us refused to leave that first day and night. The second morning our pediatrician visited and told me that we had really misbehaved and, she remarked, "Don't you realize you are fostering dependency in the child?" I responded "Dr. _____, it's obvious you have not read the literature." That did not go over big but it did get everyone off our backs. As it turned out Josh needed a second herniorraphy six months later (this had been discovered during the first surgery) and by that time we had changed pediatricians, surgeons and hospitals.

At the time of Joshua's second hospitalization I was taking a course in Interpersonal Competence with the renowned social psychologist Leonard Cottrell. He was interested in my personal experience and suggested that I do a paper for his course on "rooming-in" and use the paper to describe the theories on which I might then develop a research plan. In the process of doing this term paper I realized that this was exactly what I would study for my dissertation if nothing was going on in the field to militate against it. I corresponded with both Dr. Bowlby and James Robertson and with leading researchers in the United States whose work was related to the area of study and learned that there was no research comparing effects of hospitalization for those toddlers under standard visiting conditions and others whose parent(s) managed to stay.

It's hard to realize now that visiting privileges in pediatric units were extremely strict at that time and limited parents to as little as one or two hours a day.

The dissertation was completed in 1964 and published as a monograph by F. A. Davis in 1966. Its publication received a great deal of national attention in newspapers, magazines, and on local and national television. I was interviewed by Hugh Downs and Barbara Walters on the Today Show and received upwards of 100 letters from people telling me their own personal experiences with their children. Many of these were from hospital trustees just looking for an opportunity to influence change with data.

Ten years later I surveyed the field and was thrilled to find that major change had occurred. Clearly, the time was exactly right for change since many nurses, physicians, and parents must have been ready to move in this direction and needed an appropriate "scholarly" stimulus. It taught me a lot about the implementation of research findings into practice and the value of public relations. Without the media attention the rapid changes would not have taken place so rapidly. Also I wrote numerous articles for as many nursing journals as would accept them. Finally Martha Rogers, my boss at the Division of Nursing at NYU called me into her office and said, "Claire, don't you think you've milked this subject enough?" Well, I probably had, but for a good cause.

CHAPTER THIRTEEN

The Case for Rooming in When Young Children Are Hospitalized

Claire M. Fagin

INTRODUCTION

Hospital experiences for young children which involve separating them from their mothers have been written about extensively, talked about, and studied from a variety of aspects since 1950. It is widely recognized that the continuous and contiguous relationship of child to mothering person is essential for mentally healthy development in early childhood. Despite this, few hospitals permit mothers to remain with children during hospitalization, and some limit visiting severely. A group of investigators in England and France have been studying the response to separation when children are hospitalized. John Bowlby has described the emotional response to separation in the second and third year of life. He states, "The child becomes acutely and inconsolably distressed for a period of days, a week, or even more without a break."[1] "The immediate aftereffects, although not always evident to the trained observer, are also frequently very disquieting to the psychiatrist."[1] Roudinesco, David, and Nicolas report that "separation can have psychological effects which are sometimes permanent."[2]

Note: This was published in *Nursing Science*, August 1964.

James Robertson, in a thorough review of the literature in the area of hospitalization of children, describes the child's need for his mother being as great as his hunger for food, and believes that admitting him alone to the hospital removes from him the environment of love and security necessary to his healthy development. He goes on to say, "If, at the critical stage of early development when a young child has such a possessive and passionate need for his mother . . . he is admitted alone to a hospital . . . the child experiences a serious failure of that environment of love and security hitherto provided by his family which we know to be a necessary experience if he is to be a loving, trustful, and secure person in later life. He is too young to understand that there can be any reason . . . to justify the loss of his mother's care. . . . For, at this age, the child does not reason—he feels and he needs, and the mother he needs so intensely . . . is not there. . . . "[3]

It is widely recognized that until the child is about three years old his world revolves around his family, most particularly, about his mother. She is the essential member of the family in the fulfillment of his needs and in the delineation of his universe. The literature is unanimous in stressing the child's need for his mother, both in terms of her function in his growing personality and in his inability to comprehend termination of a separation from her. Theorists from psychobiological, instinctual, and interpersonal schools of psychiatry see the constancy of the mother-child relationship as essential in the early years of life. Piaget, after intensive study of young children, stated that "the child in extreme youth is driven to endow its parents with all of those attributes which theological doctrines assign to their divinities—sanctity, supreme power, omniscience, eternity, and even ubiquity."[4] In a later writing he pointed out that the young child has been moving from egocentricity to attributing "wholly to others the actions he can no longer consider as emanating from himself . . . he therefore invests another person with an exaggerated power over the universe."[5] The parent is thus seen as producing all events, including obviously, those involving his presence or absence. Various writers have studied children's behavior either in the hospital or after hospitalization. Robertson[3], English and Pearson[6], Gofman[7], Prugh,[8] Anna Freud,[9] and others have described the behavioral regression that many young children experience after hospitalization. English and Pearson, in describing the harmful effects of separation from the mother, discuss the events following the time when the child realizes that the mother has left him. "His development immediately ceases . . . he begins to demand that everything be done for him . . . he becomes increasingly fearful. Instead of wanting to dress, feed, and bathe himself, he acts as if he were unable to perform these routines and must have them done for him. His speech becomes more babyish. If he had ceased to suck his fingers, the habit starts again. If he had been toilet trained, he may begin to wet or soil himself. . . . "[8] Roberston describes the post-hospital behavior of young children as follows: "They sleep badly, go back on their toilet training, panic if mother goes even momentarily out of sight, and have outbursts of aggression against her."[3] There is general agreement among the authors cited on these areas.

Though many writers have recommended that mothers remain with their children during hospitalization and some hospitals permit this, there is little scientific evidence in the literature concerning the use of the mother in an effort to lessen the negative effects of the experience. Interestingly enough, in a study on reducing cross-infection among infants undergoing plastic surgery, done by the Pickerills in Australia in 1945, the mother was brought in to nurse the child.[10] Although this study was primarily concerned with cross-infection, the authors noted concomitantly that the children were happier, ate better, and gained weight. They felt that these factors also contributed to a higher resistance so infection.

At Hunterdon Medical Center in Flemington, New Jersey, mothers are encouraged to remain with their children during hospitalization. Nurses and mothers have written articles describing the program at Hunterdon in very positive terms.

Although many authors have recommended research in or utilization of the practice of mother-nursing, there is a paucity of literature concerning the latter and none concerning the former. Since no study had been done which compared the effects of the hospitalization experience itself and the effects of hospitalization when separation from the mother was an added factor, this seemed an obvious and necessary sequel to the literature in the field.

THE PROBLEM

This investigation proposed to compare selected areas of pre- and post-hospital behavior of two groups of children one and one-half through three years of age, when one group was attended by the mother during hospitalization and one group was unattended. Specifically, it was necessary to find out about (1) the behavior at the children before hospitalization; (2) the behavior of the children after hospitalization; (3) the quantity, direction, and area of change in each group; (4) the difference between the two groups; and (5) whether a relationship existed between the particular attitudes of the two groups of mothers.

THE PROCEDURE

Mothers of sixty children, one and one-half through three years of age, who were about to be hospitalized or who had just been admitted to the hospital, were interviewed before, one week after, and one month after hospitalization. Thirty of the children were semi-private or private hospital patients whose mothers remained with them during the total period of hospitalization. The other thirty children were semi-private or private hospital patients whose mothers were permitted to visit daily for a restricted period of time. Both groups of mothers wished to remain with their children. Tables 13.1 and 13.2 present the distribution of the sample with regard to age and social class. It can be seen that the groups were equivalent in those areas.

TABLE 13.1 Distribution of Sample According to Age of Children in Months

Group	X Age	t	Variance	F
Experimental	33.7		80	
		.73*		1.11*
Control	32.05		72	

*There was not a difference at the .05 level of significance in the means or variances of the two groups in age in months.

TABLE 13.2   Distribution of Sample According to Social Class of Family

Class	I	II	III	Totals
Experimental	16	7	7	30
Control	12	5	13	30
Totals	28	12	20	60
df = 2	Chi Square = 2.76[*]			

[*]This result is not significant at the .05 level.

The interview was designed to obtain information about the areas of behavior which were indicated in the literature as showing change following a separation experience. These were: dependency, reactions to temporary, brief separation; toilet training; eating habits; sleeping habits; and auto-erotic behaviors. Scales were developed to measure and compare these behaviors.

Another aspect of the study was the investigation of the mother's attitudes toward child rearing. Particular attitudes were chosen for study. These included rejection of the homemaking role, irritability, and fostering dependency. These attitudes were described by Schaefer and Bell[11] in connection with their Parental Attitude Research Instrument, PARI Final Form IV. "The scale Rejection of the Homemaking Role contains items which state the unhappiness of a woman at being shut up in a home, and her dissatisfaction with the duties of caring for the home and children. The scale Irritability was developed around items which indicate that children 'get on a woman's nerves' and that any woman would 'blow her top' frequently in the difficult job of managing a home. [the scale] . . . Fostering Dependency was designed to measure . . . [an] aspect of over-protection or over-possessiveness."[11] These attitudes were chosen in order to clarify some of the unknowns operating in the decision of the mother to stay or not to stay with her child in the hospital. For example: Did mothers who wished to remain with their children feel this way because of an unconscious wish to keep their children dependent, or was this possibly a way of compensating for rejecting attitudes toward the child? A popular notion in pediatric circles is that some mothers would do more harm than good if they remained with their children during hospitalization. In order to answer this question, the behavior of the children in both groups whose mothers obtained high scores in the negative attitudes was compared before and after hospitalization.

RESULTS OF THE STUDY

All the data were analyzed statistically, and significance of the results was determined by the use of either the *t* tests or Chi Square,[12] this depending upon the nature of the data. The results indicated very clearly that children who were not attended by the mother during hospitalization showed a significant difference between their behavior before and after hospitalization in a regressive direction. One month after hospitalization there was significant regression in the group, in reactions to temporary, brief separation from the mother (.01); emotional dependence (.001); appetite and food finickiness (.001); resistance to going to bed and sleep behavior (.05); and urine training (.01).

By contrast, the children whose mothers remained with them during the period of hospitalization did not show significant regression in their behavior but did show progressive changes in several areas. One month after hospitalization, significant differences in a progressive direction were found in reactions to temporary, brief separation; emotional dependence; appetite; manner of eating; and use of special toys. The evidence clearly indicated that when a child was not separated from his mother, his growth and development were not impeded. Indeed, some of the positive changes were dramatic. This raises questions as to the usefulness of the hospitalization as a learning experience. That is, when the mother was there supporting the youngster the anxiety generated by the experience seemed to be a spur to further maturing by the child. Additional study of this aspect is clearly implicated.

When the two groups of children were compared with each other, statistically significant results were found in reactions to temporary, brief separation from the mother (.001); emotional dependence (.001); appetite (.001); food finickiness (.001); urine training (.001); sleep behavior (.05); and manner of eating (.05). All of these were found one month after hospitalization.[*]

---

[*]Other subsidiary results were obtained, to be reported in a later publication.

In the comparison of maternal attitudes it was discovered that there was not a significant difference between the two groups of mothers in their negative attitudes toward child rearing. In addition, one-third to one-half of the mothers in each group obtained high scores in the scales Irritability and Rejection of the Homemaking Role. A separate analysis was done of their children's pre- and post-hospital behavior. It was found that there were no significant regressive differences for the children in the experimental group while there were significant regressive differences for the children in the control group. This further confirmed the findings and gave evidence that they were independent of maternal attitude. No high scores were found among mothers in either group in the scale Fostering Dependency. These results cast doubt on the notions that some mothers would do more harm than good if they remained with their children during hospitalization and that mothers who do remain wish unconsciously to keep their children dependent.

CONCLUSION

It is apparent that children who are one and one-half through three years old react with regressive behavior to a hospital experience which involves separation from the mother. Despite the traumatic nature of surgical procedures and other hospital treatments, children hospitalized with the mother present do not show regressive behaviors following hospitalization. In fact, positive changes in behavior were reported (often with surprise) by the mother.

It is important to recognize that this study was limited to white families whose socioeconomic status was middle class and above. It would be valuable to extend the findings to a larger sphere. It is interesting to note that some of the hospitals which permit mothers to room in on the semi-private and private floors have restricted visiting on the ward. It would seem in some cases that the theories of child development apply only to those who (1) are acquainted with these theories and (2) can afford to carry them out. One wonders whether this particular kind of trauma is limited by socioeconomic class.

The results of this study clearly suggest the need to increase the visiting privileges for mothers when young children are hospitalized.

Nursing personnel and physicians should not view this as a special favor to parents but should understand that the attendance of the mother is necessary for the mental health of the child. Not only should mothers be permitted to remain with their children, they should be encouraged to do so. This implies changes in attitudes as well as in the roles which nurses and doctors fulfill. Encouraging the mother to become a participant in the hospital experience implies accepting and seeking to understand her feelings as well as those of the child. It also implies planning with and assisting the parent in order to maximize her participation in caring for the child. Although initially these aspects may appear to be time consuming, the investment of time should tend to free nursing personnel once the mother's orientation is completed. Practitioners of medicine and nursing, working as partners, could eliminate or greatly reduce the traumatic features of hospitalization for young children.

> "Remember, opponents of social change always urge delay because of some present crisis."
>
> —Wendell Wilkie

ENDNOTES

1. Bowlby, J. (1952). Maternal Care and Mental Health (194 pp. 23, 25). World Health Organization, Geneva.
2. Roudinesco, J., David, M., & Nicholas, J. (1952). Responses of Young Children to Separation from their Mothers. Courrier du Centre International de l'Enface, II: 66.
3. Robertson, J. (1958). *Young children in hospitals.* New York: Basic Books.
4. Piaget, J. (1929). *The child's conception of the world* (p. 378). Routledge and Kegan Paul Ltd., London.
5. Piaget, J. (1954). *The construction of reality in the child* (p. 308). New York: Basic Books.
6. English, O., Spurgeon, & Pearson, G. (1945). *Emotional Problems of Living* (pp. 34–95). New York: Norton Co.
7. Gofman, H., Buckman, W., & Schade, G. H. (1957). The Child's Emotional Response to Hospitalization. *American Medical Association Journal Disability of Children, 93,* 157–163.
8. Prugh, D. et al. (1953). A Study of the Emotional Reactions of Children and Families to Hospitalization. *American Journal Orthopsychiatry, 23,* 70–106.

9. Freud, A. (1952). The Role of Bodily Illness in the Mental Life of Children. *Psychoanalytic Study of the Child, VII,* 69–82.

10. Pickerill, C. M., & H. P. (1954). Elimination of Hospital Cross-infection in Children-nursing by the Mother. *Lancet, I,* 425–429.

11. Schaefer, E. S., & Bell, R. Q. (1958). Development of a Parental Attitude Research Instrument. *Child Development, 29*(3), 339–361.

12. Downey, N. M., & Heath, R. W. (1959). *Basic statistical methods* (p. 136). New York: Harper and Brothers.

PART FOUR

Looking Ahead

CHAPTER FOURTEEN

Y2K: Nurses Can Turn on the Heat in Health Care

Claire M. Fagin

"**B**e of good cheer, the world has never yet witnessed any great revolution which was not brought about gradually, sometimes almost imperceptibly. In proof of this we have only to look backward over the history of our own profession . . . we stand today upon the attainments of our predecessors, and our gathering here is proof that we realize how much yet remains to be accomplished." Nursing leader Mary Agnes Snively (1893) gave us this advice more than 100 years ago.

Snively believed that what appear to be radical changes are not always as overwhelming or rapid as they seem. Historical precedents more often follow her rule than not, although in our nation we have seen overwhelming radical change in some arenas, such as the introduction of Social Security and later Medicare, for example, and currently the domination of for-profit companies in health service delivery. Actually our fee for service medical care system was always for-profit but with the exception of pharmaceutical companies the profits were kept by the providers rather than put in the pockets of

Note: This chapter is an edited version of an address to the New York State Nurses Association, October 14, 1999, Lake Placid, New York.

Wall Street investors. The current state of affairs is not a happy one for nurses, hospitals, and physicians, and it is my view that the early years of the 21st century will bring a reversal in this trend. What we need to do now as we reflect on our progress and possibilities, is to use our strengths to develop strategies for change that protect our patients, and our nurses, and provide the environment for attracting the next generation of nurses—perhaps the most important danger we face at this time.

The women who formed the template for nursing's current organizations over a century ago didn't have the vote, had few property rights, and had precious few career opportunities available to them, but these women were anything but powerless victims of second class citizenship. On the contrary, they were highly regarded, influential citizens who helped develop every aspect of our health care system—from safe hospitals, to home and community care, to social services, to obstetrics and pediatrics, and more.

Today, on the other hand, women vote, have property rights and ever expanding career horizons. So it is all the more ironic that from the nursing executive to the staff nurse, nurses are being "disappeared" from many parts of our health care modalities.

Perhaps one of the reasons for the disappearing nurse is that nurses see too much. With its hints of omniscience and advocacy, nursing is increasingly threatening to the powers that be. With our commitment to care, and omniscient position in observing the flaws and foibles of individuals and organizations in health care, some administrators and managers have the hope that we can again become subservient and invisible.

But that won't happen. Nursing leadership has come of age and now, at the beginning of a new millennium we have the opportunity, not to say the imperative, to bring this leadership to bear on what should be our top priority: Universal health care. This presentation will discuss the public's concerns about the current state of health care, the flaws in current approaches and some solutions we can offer by again coalescing around the development of a strong public movement for a universal health care system.

THE NATURE OF PUBLIC CONCERNS

I want to start this discussion with a short summary of the nature of public concerns. I start here because it is clear that unless we and others can mobilize public interest there is little hope for the kind of change that we believe vital in health care. The fact is, there is considerable conflict in reports about the concerns of the public. Some surveys tell us that the public is unhappy and frightened about what may happen to them if they get sick. Other surveys tell us that the public is generally satisfied with health and medical care and with the services of their HMOs. For example, in Blendon's 1990 international survey,[2] we learned that Americans were very dissatisfied with health care and that among the ten nations surveyed only Italians were as dissatisfied. In more recent surveys we see the ambivalence our fellow citizens have always shown to government intervention. The 1998 Kaiser/Harvard/PSRA survey[3] found that while a majority of Americans favored government regulation of managed care even if it increased cost, most insured Americans were satisfied with their health insurance plan. Those most in favor of regulation were those who described their own health as poor, only fair, or good, and had some college education. Those who identified themselves as Republicans, and in self-described excellent or very good health were least in favor of government regulation. Even with this sense of satisfaction, a majority of Americans expressed concern that they might not receive the services they need when they are very sick. Recognize that 80% of Americans do not use health services in any given year.

One survey reported in 1999[4] shows widespread discontent with the U.S. health system with only one of six Americans supporting the status quo. One third of the adults surveyed said the health care system should be rebuilt.

THE CONTRADICTIONS IN PUBLIC CONCERNS

The conflicts in what we hear about public concerns regarding health care are important to understand if we are to develop effective strategies to promote universal health care. I have promoted nurse/consumer collaboration for many years. Reviewing the events of this decade have disillusioned me mightily in this regard. I had believed that with full disclosure of information consumers could and would play an active, informed part in the reform of health care. Two of our assumptions were: 1. People know what's best for themselves, and 2. people will make choices that are in their best interest when there is sufficient information available. Both wrong. In health care people may not *always* know what is best for themselves even with a barrage of information. Secondly, even if they do, their choices are not necessarily in their best interest. Think of smoking, obesity, use of addictive substances, and many more behavioral indicators that the rules of the informed consumer many of us cherish do not work, necessarily. Clearly, this goes for health reform. Health care consumers are more likely to rely on personal experiences or the recommendations of friends and family members than on research, report cards, and the like. Unless there is a constant barrage of negative news coverage, issues do not emerge as part of the public's policy agenda.

Part of any plan for universal health care must deal with the problem of the uninsured. Although health care reform did not rank among voters' top five in the surveys I mentioned, the problem of the uninsured did rank high in voters' concerns. Thirty-three percent said it was the most important health care reform goal, followed by 27% who said that making health care more affordable was the most important goal. Forty-seven percent said that government action should be taken on the issue of the uninsured even if new taxes were required. By a margin of 74% to 19%, voters said they would be more likely to vote for a Member of Congress who makes affordable health care a priority over tougher HMO regulations.

While the ambivalence of the public towards overall reform is clear, the most recent Commonwealth Survey (1998) pointed to the value placed on quality of care and access and the public's fears that quality of care may be eroding. This fear is leading to high anxiety and support for change. The public has expressed fear about care in hospitals, even if they have not yet had a personal experience. The fear is that nurses will not be available to care for them. All surveys rank nurses as highest on the public's list of trusted persons, and, of course, with fears of sickness and hospitalization, the threat of a shortage of nurses caused by profit taking and cutbacks looms large. So far in this decade nursing has been both extremely active and seriously under-represented in discussions about a universal health care system. In present discussions about universal health care some nursing organizations have joined with the Ad Hoc Committee to Protect Health Care, and the Nurses Network for a National Health Plan to endorse some form of single payer system. Nurses are less visible in other groups and given the extent to which nurses are trusted, we have the potential to be extremely powerful both in discussions about health care reform and in discussions about patients rights in managed care. Before it is too late, the public's trust in nursing must be exploited in the service of fundamental systemic change.

In June of 1999 the nation's seven largest physician groups announced a grassroots effort to challenge Congress and year 2000 presidential candidates to make universal health care coverage their top election priority. The seven groups (the American Medical Association, American Academy of Family Physicians, American Academy of Pediatrics, American College of Emergency Physicians, American College of Obstetricians and Gynecologists, American College of Physicians-American Society of Internal Medicine, and American College of Surgeons) vowed to ensure that all Americans have health care coverage, that policies include quality benefit packages and that medical necessity decisions "reflect generally accepted standards of medical practice." One reporter commented, "If you add up all the doctors in all the medical groups that are supporting this political effort, it comes to more than 600,000 . . . affluent professionals—pillars of their communities . . . who cannot be dismissed as leftists or uninformed dreamers."[5]

These groups and others need *us* to be part of their coalitions, but nurses as a group must also stand alone with strong visibility in order to capitalize on the trust which the public has in us. Whether or not the public is ready, or unconflicted, we must be ready to get behind political candidates with our own plan, that has, at least, the support of all of our nursing organizations and many other colleagues. We did this before in 1993 and were unbelievably successful in developing a nurses' national health plan which well over 40 organizations endorsed. We have the power to do this again and the timing could not be better.

FLAWS IN CURRENT APPROACHES

There are so many flaws in current approaches that I will only summarize them briefly and focus on the mismatch between the

Wall Street approach and health care. When nursing organizations coalesced around a plan for universal health care we saw managed care as the organizing philosophy of that care. Since the term managed care is being used to describe the market manipulation of cost it is a distortion of what we and others had in mind. Despite problems identified daily, many congressman and Senators, and no less an august figure than Alan Greenspan, state their belief in the market system and join with insurers opposed to regulation or restraint on market practices. Managed care industry contentions not withstanding, a yet-to-be-released report from the GAO says that Medicare is still overpaying HMOs despite cuts under the 1997 Balanced Budget Act. The industry has been walking out of the Medicare business at the same time that they continue aggressive efforts to attract older people. They have left many stranded across the country. Yet as I have said, there are still many who believe that the market paradigm is appropriate in health care even though it follows few rules of the market. Remember, the sine qua non of market discipline is that people can vote with their feet when they don't like the product. Even where choice is available, users are unable to choose on the basis of quality since quality indicators are largely unavailable.

Consumer Reports rated HMOs according to which their readers liked best. The plans at the top of their list were all not-for-profit HMOs with years of experience. Most of the poor performers were for-profit HMOs and many of the lower ranked plans refused to reveal data on how well they satisfy their members. Readers who said they were ill were generally less satisfied . . . than other respondents. Only 33% of those readers were completely or very satisfied.[6]

Furthermore, a study published in the summer of 1999 found that "patients enrolled in profit-making health insurance plans are significantly less likely to receive the basics of good medical care" than their counterparts in not-for-profit HMOs. This study has earned the ire of the insurance industry. Himmelstein, Woolhandler, Hellander, and Wolfe compared care in 248 for-profit and 81 non-profit health plans across the country that provided medical care for 56% of all Americans enrolled in HMOs in 1996. The study found that compared with not-for-profit plans, for-profit HMOs scored lower on 14 quality measures, including four of the most important preventive care measures, childhood immunizations, routine mammograms,

Pap smears, prenatal care, and beta-blockers treatment for heart attack patients.[7]

The growth in the uninsured is proof positive of the failure of the market model to reform the health care system. Maybe the market can trim costs and improve efficiency for customers in other fields. But by definition the uninsured are not customers—they aren't paying if they aren't buying. Other industries are not required to supply non-customers, but health care is not just another industry. In health care the uninsured have to matter to us. Unavailability of preventive and primary care bodes ill for the uninsured and for all of us whose costs are increased when uncompensated care equates to care of the seriously ill. All Americans will get sick someday and will all need care. If not sooner than later and if later care will be needed longer and it will be more expensive.

As a New Yorker I have a big stake in this population of the uninsured. New York State has a higher proportion of uninsured than the country at large and New York City has an even higher proportion. In the nation, about 16% of the population is uninsured, in New York State it's 17% and in New York City one of every four residents is uninsured—a whopping 25%.[8] Experts like the United Hospital Fund of New York agree that one of the main factors in the growth of the uninsured is the steady erosion in private insurance coverage we have witnessed over the past decade; again worse in New York State than in the rest of the country. In 1990, more than 73% of New Yorkers and Americans in general were offered private health insurance by their employers. By 1996 that percentage for Americans was reduced to 70%, and for New Yorkers only 65% had private coverage. This picture is continuing to worsen at a time of a booming economy, a very healthy New York, and a reduction in the rate of growth of health expenditures.

Interestingly, Governor George Pataki has announced a health care package that offers coverage to thousands of uninsured New Yorkers and helps pay for it by boosting the tax on cigarettes.[8] The package expands the child health program to adults and would cover about 180,000 adults over the next few years.

There are so many misconceptions about the uninsured that it is worth spending a few more minutes on this population. First, two-thirds of the uninsured are working; about 12% work part time. While they are disproportionately low income, most are above the poverty line—most of those below the poverty line qualify for public programs like Medicaid. While many suffer from chronic illness or are at risk medically the group as a whole is disproportionately in need of fewest health services. The uninsured are most often between the ages of 19 and 34—an age group actuaries love because they rarely show up in the hospital. In New York City, 35% of residents in the childbearing group are uninsured, compared with only 13% of residents age 50–64. Among Hispanics, the group most likely to be uninsured, more than half of all 20-somethings are uninsured. Some 11MM of the uninsured are children under 18 years of age.

So the profile of the uninsured in New York is a low income working person, often young, often Hispanic.

The government and we the public have become hostages to employers and insurers in health care. Right now the United States spends 14.2% of our GNP on health services, as contrasted to Canada's 9.2%. As I mentioned earlier, even the Health Insurance Association of America's survey told us that 47% of voters said that government action should be taken on the issue of the uninsured even if new taxes were required. If the 2 million increase we saw this year becomes the norm, just think of the public's reaction.

(SO WHAT ARE) OUR SOLUTIONS

In 1993 when all of our organizations supported a nurses' national health plan we defined several ingredients for a successful health service future that would serve all Americans. We called for a pay or play system, a system which would rely on managing care and on outcome evaluations, consumer empowerment through full disclosure and choice of providers, protections against over-treatment, and incrementalism starting with pregnant women, infants and children.

We had lots of good stuff in our 1993 plan but it needs a tuning up so that it reflects our learning and the current political/health care climate. Clearly, neither pay or play nor incrementalism resonates now. With over 44 MM of our population uninsured, (many employed) it is clear that a solution must be found immediately for this problem. Pay or play is not so attractive as it was because in this 6 year period the insurance picture for the insured has changed dramatically and can be expected to change even more. In this decade we will find that employment and health benefits will not be linked as they were in the past. We are seeing many signs of this at present as more and more people are involved in shorter term jobs, contract employment, and the like. Some companies are considering eliminating completely segmented benefits and giving employees lump sums from which employees can choose just which benefits they want. The problem of the uninsured is coupled with the failure or shortcomings of the Kennedy-Kassebaum solution. The General Accounting Office of the Congress has told us that people who exercise their rights under the law are often charged premiums far higher than standard rates. One insurer said it reserved the right to charge high-risk individuals five times the rates charged to healthy people.

For pay or play to work the country must strengthen the system with a mandate that all employers must cover workers. Given the changes in employment we are seeing, even if a mandate were possible it would not take care of the problem. Richard Hinkel, a senior analyst at the Wisconsin Insurance Commissioner's Office, predicts "double-digit" rate increases for the year 2000. Business leaders see this as an employee issue because "employees are being asked to absorb more and more of these costs." Wisconsin business owner Fred Honkamp, whose company went from a plan in which employees paid no out-of-pocket expenses to one that required co-pays and deductibles, said, "We're bracing for our next contract . . . I don't know if we can afford to have health insurance at all." This is going to be a recurrent theme. So much for pay or play.

It should be clear to all of us that a universal system will not be feasible without managing care. But as I said in an earlier chapter, nurses have always believed that *managing care is an appropriate concept* which addresses the problems of a fragmented and disease oriented fee for service system with disincentives for cost constraint. In reaction to those problems however, we have gotten an inappropriate, for-profit managed cost system where unconstrained profit incentives have brought us to the crisis of today. Managed care was supposed to "bring about organized health care systems in which doctors and managers would be working hard to improve the quality and cut the costs," says Alain Enthoven, one of the original "fathers of managed care." But the fact is that managed care promised too much and has delivered too little."[9]

The issue of consumer choice which we stressed in 1993, is, as the Ad Hoc Committee states, "the foundation of patient autonomy." Choices of providers, hospitals, home care agencies and nursing homes, and other modalities of care are important for the empowered consumer. People need the freedom to seek second or at times even third or fourth opinions and they must have enough choice to form relationships with someone they trust. Trust is a sine qua non of the relationship between clinician and patient. How do you build trust without time to develop a relationship and listen to what the patient is saying? All health providers and patients are suffering from the lack of time and the building of trust and physicians as well as nurses are seeing this problem as increasing and extremely serious. So choice alone, (without appropriate time) will not solve the problem of a trusting relationship with the provider chosen.

The notion of outcome evaluations as a requisite to appropriate care has not been exercised even where studies are available. Both over-treatment and inappropriate treatment are still problems. A study conducted by Rand showed hysterectomies performed for inappropriate reasons, bountiful prescribing of antibiotics for colds, insufficient immunizations for the elderly, and acceptance of medical advances before "substantial knowledge of benefits and risks has accumulated."[10] Furthermore, surveys about quality of care in hospitals and HMOs are not worth the paper they use. The designs are faulty, and an increasing number of organizations are refusing or are delinquent in submitting completed documents. The issue of outcomes is an important one and better methodology as well as strategies for appropriate mandates should be part of our proposal for a universal health system. Managing care must rely on the state of the art in outcome evaluation.

In our 1993 plan we talked about the centrality of nurses in managing care. That of course must remain our key plank. Nurses are a chief means of containing costs while providing quality care that affords universal access. We all know by now that nurse practitioners and clinical nurse specialists can lower costs, and improve quality of care and access to care.[11] Where legal and reimbursement constraints restricted nurse practitioners' potential in the past this is no longer true in most states in the country. It is remarkable that nursing has achieved what seemed like an impossible dream just a few years ago.

Nursing expertise is at the heart of preventive, primary, and home care services. Nurses can manage the challenge of cost containment and show the experience of all too many years being the only ones to take the issue seriously. Nurses are patient advocates who know how to manage care because that is what all nursing is whether in or out of hospital. There is no way for nurses to juggle 2, 4, 6, 8, or today sometimes 18 patients without managing the care that they give. Nurses put the interests of the patient first, prioritize care, and try to put the bottom line second. I believe the true interests of patients are cost effective as well. Giving the appropriate treatment, at the appropriate time is an example of good care and care that will reduce costs in the near and long term. Managed care organizations are not patient advocates. Rather they are advocates for the private sector marketplace, and all too often lack the knowledge for the clinical judgments they are making. By reducing care but not inappropriate treatment, by reducing nurses' roles in hospitals, by treating patients with high-tech treatments but ill-trained carers, care will ultimately be not only ineffective but inefficient and more costly to the system and to the individual patient.

Nurses cannot be passive observers now or in the future. We cannot allow things to just happen to us and the patients we serve. We remain the lifeline of patients and their families as they experience the changes of the health care system. Yet being a lifeline, when many of us see ourselves as powerless in the large health policy scene, can be frustrating and enervating. The challenge of control becomes a crucial component as we try to deal with patients' problems. Nursing is at a turning point with regard to this dimension.

But, not only are *we* at a turning point. With us at this chaotic time is the public, ever more vulnerable, as they see themselves more and more as powerless victims of change. We know about these feelings of powerlessness from phone calls for help when health and illness troubles hit people we know or their friends and families. As the population ages a greater proportion of people will have exposure to the sickness care system. We need to work with the public on a large scale through specialty-based, disease-centered advocacy groups, and on smaller scales in all our professional and social contacts. We need to explain what is happening and why to patients and families. The public and the media are willing and ready to listen to health care workers who marshal their facts, use appropriate studies and tell compelling stories. The problem is not enough of us do this. And there was never a better time, when public confidence in nurses is at an all time high. Achieving the public trust is not a small thing and we must use this privileged position responsibly and to the fullest.

To help us move our agenda forward, I believe the major national initiative to accomplish our ultimate aim—universal health, should focus on the States. I join Suzanne Gordon and Alan Sager at the Boston University School of Public Health in thinking that the most effective way to bring our vision to the public in this political climate is to place our energy at the state level. First then, while we must make health care part of the debate in all political campaigns, more realistically, part of the national movement to be created would encourage and support state initiatives. It is evident that without some national crisis it is unrealistic to seek national Congressional action. Second, a coordinating national group could help target states in which there are political groups, union groups, and advocacy groups that can help design legislation, referenda, or both. This national group will help state groups design model legislation and answer the 50 to 100 important questions about the design of the system. They will also have to be prepared to deal with and gain federal support for ERISA and Medicare and Medicaid waivers. Third, the national group would develop appropriate coalitions to share information and arguments, strategies and tactics so that we do not reinvent the wheel every two or three weeks. Fourth, studies need to be conducted of the costs, coverage, quality, and savings of universal health care in states experimenting with particular models. Alan Sager and his colleagues conducted such a study in Massachusetts. The study informs the design of the legislation and details how to raise the money, how to contain costs, how to pay hospitals, doctors, nurses, and other health care workers, how to provide long term care, and mental health care. These studies, done state by state, will show how to save money, how to cut administrative and clinical fat, and how to expand benefits for currently insured people and the uninsured. Fifth, the national coalition group should stimulate states to run referenda to build support for legislation and help to create compelling arguments to promote the legislation. And finally, number six is organizing, organizing, organizing. Because of the way nursing is organized we are in a powerful position to foster the national movement.

As proposals are made, we need to evaluate all of them on grounds of inclusiveness, appropriate coverage, access, and quality indicators. But as nurses we also need to evaluate proposals on some of the "C" words we cherish. Does the proposal reflect compassion for those who suffer, does it value and empower communities and people in them, and is it courageous enough to confront the root causes of our nation's health problems?

One strategy for defining and maintaining our compassion while recognizing and adapting to the cost problems of the current situation is to keep our focus always on the patient in the changing health and medical care scene. When we look at what works and what doesn't, the object of that examination should be the effects on patient care. Clarity about the pluses and minuses of change will inevitably involve nurses and nursing care but as a secondary rather than a primary focus. Maintaining the primary focus on the patient reflects a maturing profession with compassion as its byword. It also reflects a growing sense of community.

Where health care is concerned the notion of community also makes economic sense. Health costs go up when people lack access to primary care, to prenatal care, where children are not immunized, and where the public is uninformed.

But policymakers have not always approached health care as a community issue. Health care is such a personal experience, Americans are tempted to view it exclusively as a personal problem—a problem facing individuals, not society as a whole. Challenges like AIDS, tuberculosis, and sexually transmitted diseases have heightened our awareness over the past decade that health is a community's problem.

No one can address health care reform without the third "C"— *courage.* The time for courage is just starting and I suspect the need for courage will escalate in the coming few years. It will take persistent courage to press for, and continue to press for, the changes we as nurses know to be essential to successful reform as well as to monitor the effects of changes, such as restructuring on patient care.

In conclusion let me state five points of specific advice:

1—Know what you are doing and be able to articulate it to audiences other than these individuals with nursing; control what comes out of your mouth when you are talking about nursing; do not allow yourself to get into the new corporate lingo of calling sick people customers, or business partners. Speak clearly, in language both you and the patient and family and all your non-nursing contacts can understand.

2—Support your colleagues in their goal of quality patient care; when they or you stand alone of course there is risk and impotence; when you stand together you are safer, feel really good about your position, and, as long as you are talking about patient care, no one can doubt your public interest. Speak up as you hear your colleagues individually speak for patient care. Pressure the nursing executives in your organizations to constantly remember that they are nurses.

3—Recognize the importance and reputation of nurses with the public and use this importance. Don't waste it!

4—Be active in the current debates in Congress and with the candidates for national office. Whichever of the candidates you support make sure that they have a health platform that includes a strategy for achieving universal health. As I said we need to refocus our major attention on state plans which can serve as an impetus to the nation and meet at least the needs of the insured and uninsured of our own state.

5—Wrestle together to find solutions to problems—join with the advocacy groups which have organized to defend health care. Our own Nurses Network for a National Health Program is a good place to start. This group has been endorsed by the New York State Nurses Association and is an active part of a national, interdisciplinary effort. We need to evaluate what others are doing at the same time that we work on our own proposals. In that way we can negotiate for our preferences with our collaborating organizations.

Remembering always the vision, goals, and values that brought us to this field we must use our expertise and knowledge in providing and safeguarding quality patient care. We cannot afford to shortchange care which will eventually backfire on us and on patients. We cannot afford to step aside quietly and give others an exclusive forum to present reduced nurse/patient ratios as satisfactory and harmless. Health care quality is the raison d'être for professionalism. We must uphold the autonomy and professionalism of the nursing role, but recognize that autonomy is not lost in partnership with the public and other colleagues.

As we move into the 21st century it's time to create a genuine health care system that balances care and cure, and recognizes the extraordinary accomplishments of this past century. It's time to turn up the heat in the year 2000, so *we* can work in a health care system *that works* and in which our *patients* can benefit fully from our achievements.

ENDNOTES

1. Snively, M. A. (1893). Address to first convention of National League for Nursing (original name: American Society of Superintendents of Training Schools for Nurses).
2. Blendon, R. J., et al. (1990). Satisfaction with health systems in ten nations. *Health Affairs, 9,* 2, 185–192.
3. Blendon, R. J., et al. (1998). Understanding the managed care backlash. *Health Affairs, 17,* 4.
4. Commonwealth Fund 1998 International Health Policy Survey. (1999). *Health Affairs,* May/June.
5. Cocco, M. (1999, August 26). OpEd. *Newsday.*
6. Lieberman, T. (1999, August). How does your HMO stack up? *Consumer Reports.*
7. Stolberg (1999, July 14). *The New York Times.*
8. Communication from Leah Binder, Mayor's Office. August 25, 1999.
9. American Health Line. September 19, 1999.
10. Greenberg, D. (1999, July 13). How Good is the Quality of Health Care in the United States? *Journal of Commerce.*
11. Office of Technology Assessment. Physician assistants and certified nurse-midwives: A policy analysis, a p. 6, b p. 66, Washington DC, Government Printing Office, 1986 (plus many subsequent studies).

Index

Page numbers followed by t indicate table. Pages numbers followed by f indicate figure.